Fu Qing-zhu's Formula Book on Men's Diseases

Fù Qīng Zhǔ Nán Kē

傅 青 主 男 科

Fu Qing-zhu

Translators:

Hongzhan Zhao

Xianhui Zhang

Fu Qing-zhu's Formula Book on Men's Diseases

ISBN:	Softcover	978-1-4836-2168-5
	Ebook	978-1-4836-2169-2

Rev. date: 04/09/2013

To order additional copies of this book, contact:
Xlibris Corporation
1-800-618-969
www.Xlibris.com.au
Orders@Xlibris.com
503570

Acknowledgement

I am pleased to acknowledge the assistance of many people in the preparation of this book. First of all, we have benefited from the help and advice of Mr. Jonathan Schell with TCM Database, U.S.A., who has guided the process of initial translation, reviewed this book repeatedly and provided detailed suggestions for translation.

The staffs at Shandong TCM College are exceptionally helpful, and we are especially grateful to these people: Dr. Jing Zheng, Dr. Jiang Xia, Dr. Wang Dawei of TCM Department; Mr. Shen Wei, Mr. Song Lei of Medicine Department for lending their expertise to the translation.

Finally, I want to thank my family members, for their understanding and accepting our physical and mental absence from our family life during the past five years of translation.

Hongzhan Zhao

2013-2-3

Contents

Fu Qing-zhu's Formula Book on Men's Diseases

Fù Qīng Zhǔ Nán Kē

傅青主男科

Book I

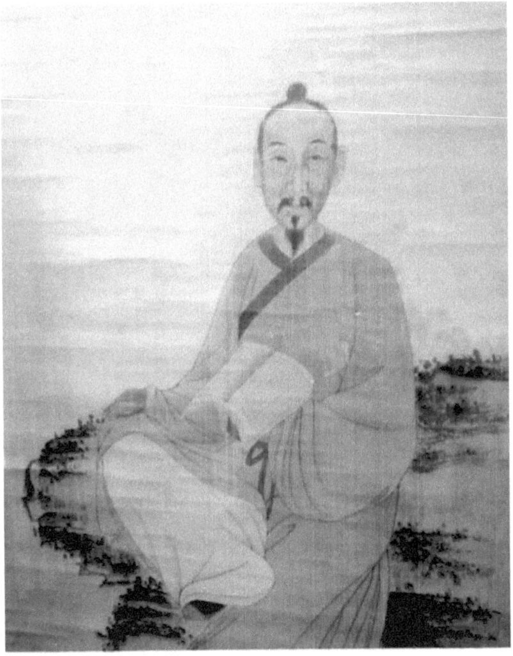

A portrait of Fu Qingzhu

傷寒門

Chapter 1 Cold Damage

初病說

凡病初起之時，用藥原易奏功。無如世人看不清症，用藥錯亂，往往致變症蜂起；苟看病清，用藥當，何變症之有？

On Onset of Diseases

On onset, any disease is easily medicated. However, common practitioners can hardly differentiate symptoms clearly, and the medicines they wrongly administered often cause swarms of deterioration to rise. If the disease had been diagnosed and medicated properly, how could the deterioration have risen?

傷風

按古方書皆曰中風，今曰傷風。

凡人初傷風，必然頭痛身痛，咳嗽痰多，鼻流清水，切其脈必浮。方用：荊芥、防風、柴胡、黃芩、半夏、甘草各等分，水煎服，一劑即止，不必再劑也。

Wind Damage

It is called "wind-stroke" in all ancient formulae books, but named as *"wind damage"*[1] nowadays.

On onset, patients of wind damage invariably have symptoms of headache, generalized pain, cough with profuse phlegm, runny noses with clear watery discharge, and patients' pulses must be *floating*[2] if taken. Formula for wind damage consists of equal amount of the following medicinals:

荊芥	jīng jiè	Leaf of Schizonepeta tenuifolia
防風	fang fēng	Root of Ledebouriella divaricata
柴胡	chái hú	Root of Bupleurum chinense
黃芩	huáng qín	Root of Scutellaria baicalensis
半夏	bàn xià	Rhizome of Pinellia ternata
甘草	gān cǎo	Root of Glycyrrhiza uralensis

[1] *wind damage:* this may also be referred to as *wind invasion*, which is interpreted in modern times as the "common cold".

[2] *floating pulse*: a superficially located pulse which can be felt by light touch and grows faint on hard pressure.

One dose of *water decoction*[3] will do, no more dose is needed.

傷寒

凡傷寒初起，鼻塞目痛，項強頭痛，切其脈必浮緊。方用：桂枝、乾葛、陳皮、甘草各等分。水煎服，一劑即愈。

Cold Damage

On onset, *cold damage*[4] has symptoms of nasal congestion, eye pain, headache with rigid neck, and invariably floating and *tight pulse*[5]. Formula for cold damage consists of equal amount of:

桂枝 guì zhī Twigs of Cinnamonum cassia

---

[3] *water decoction*: Decoction is a method for extraction by boiling herbal or other materials to extract chemical substances.*Unless otherwise stipulated, all other formulae are intended for water decoction.*

[4] *cold damage*: (1) a general term for various externally contracted febrile diseases; (2) a condition caused by cold, manifested as chills and fever, absence of sweating, headache, and floating tense pulse.

[5] *tight pulse*: a pulse that feels like a tightly stretched cord.

乾葛	gān gē	Root of Pueraria lobata
陳皮	chén pí	Peel of Citrus reticulata
甘草	gān cǎo	Root of Glycyrrhiza uralensis

Water decoctin. One dose cures.

外感

外感之發熱，衛氣外閉也；內傷之發熱，營氣內損也；外感熱在皮毛，內傷熱在骨髓，治法不同。外感發熱方見下。凡人外感，必然發熱。方用：

柴胡、黃芩、荊芥、半夏、甘草各等分，水煎服。

四時不正之氣，來犯人身，必然由皮毛而入榮衛。故用柴胡、荊芥，先散皮毛之邪，邪既先散，安得入內？又有半夏以袪痰，使邪不得挾痰以作祟；黃芩以清火，使邪不得挾火以作殃，甘草調藥以和中，是以邪散而無傷於正氣也。若內傷之發熱，則不可用此方。

External Contraction

Fever of *external contraction*[6] is the result of external

[6] *external contraction*: a disease or morbid condition produced by any of the six excesses (external etiological factors) or other noxious factors, the same as exopathic disease.

blockage of defensive qi4, while fever of internal damage is the result of internal damage of nutrient qi4. In case of the former, fever affects patient's *skin and body hair*[7]; As to the latter, fever affects the *marrow*[8]. Therefore, their therapies should be different. A formula for externally contracted fever is stipulated here-in-after. The external contraction is invariably symptomized with increased body temperature. Formula is equal amount of:

柴胡	chái hú	Root of Bupleurum chinense
黄芩	huáng qín	Root of Scutellaria baicalensis
荊芥	jīng jiè	Leaf of Schizonepeta tenuifolia
半夏	bàn xià	Rhizome of Pinellia ternate
甘草	gān cǎo	Root of Glycyrrhiza uralensis

When pathogenic factors of the four seasons attack, they invariably penetrate into the circulation of blood and the movement of defensive qi4 through patient's skin and body hair. Therefore, **chái hú** and **jīng jiè** are employed to

---

[7] *skin and body hair*: a collective term for skin and its fine hair.

[8] *marrow*: an extraordinary organ including bone marrow and spinal marrow, both of which are nourished by the kidney essence.

disperse pathogens from the skin and body hair. How can the evils enter human body since they have been dispersed? **Bàn xià** dispels phlegm in order that the pathogens are refrained from becoming a courier combining with phlegm; **Huáng qín** clears fire so that pathogens can do no harm by taking fire with them; **Gān cǎo** coordinates the medicinals, and harmonizes the center and middle energizer. As a result, those pathogens are all dispersed and can do no harm to the *upright qi4*[9]. This formula is not applicable to fever of internal damage.

傷食

凡傷食必心中飽悶，見食則惡，食之轉痛也。方用：

白朮、茯苓、枳殼各壹錢、穀芽、麥芽各貳錢、山楂貳拾箇、神麴伍錢、半夏壹錢、甘草伍分、砂仁參粒。

水煎服，一劑快，二劑愈。

Food Damage

[9] *Upright qi4*: also known as *zheng qi4* or *healthy qi4*, it is a collective designation for the normal functions of human body and the abilities to maintain health, including the abilities of self-regulation, adaptation.

Symptoms of *Food Damage*[10] are stomach fullness with depression, aversion to food and stomachache after food intake. Formula:

白朮	bái zhú	Rhizome of Atractylodes macrocephala	1*qian*[11]
茯苓	fú líng	Dried fungus of Poria cocos	1 qian
枳殼	zhǐ ké	Dried peel of Aurantii Fructus	1 qian
穀芽	gǔ yá	Sprout of Oryza sativa	2 qian
麥芽	mài yá	Fruit of Hordei Germinatus	2 qian
山楂	shān zhā	Fruit of Crateagus pinnatifida	20 pieces
神麴	shén qū	Medicated leaven	5 qian
半夏	bàn xià	Rhizome of Pinellia ternata	1 qian
甘草	gān cǎo	Root of Glycyrrhiza uralensis	5 *fen*[12]
砂仁	shā rén	Fruit of Amomum villosum	3 pieces

The first dose inhibits and the second cures.

---

[10] *Food Damage*: any disease which damages the spleen and stomach due to food.

[11] *qian*: a weight unit of ancient China, one qian equals 3.125 grams.

[12] *fen*: a weight unit of ancient China, 1 qian = 10 fen, 1 fen = 0.3125 gram.

瘧疾方用遇仙丹

此方丸之大小，未曾定分兩。愚酌以壹錢為凖，南方之人，以及老弱久瘧，尤宜減半：

生軍陸兩，檳榔、三稜、莪朮、黑醜、白醜各參兩，木香貳兩，甘草壹兩，水丸。

遇發日清晨，溫水化三、四丸，尋以溫米飲補之。忌生冷、魚腥、蕎麵，孕婦勿服。

Yuxian Pills: A Sovereign Remedy for Malaria

The unit weight is not specified originally in this formula. From my humble point of view, one qian per pill is the standard weight. It is more appropriate to take half-qian pills for Southerners, elders, impotent people, and those sufferers of chronic malaria. Formula:

生軍	shēng jūn	Root of Rheum palmatum	6 liang
檳榔	bīng láng	Fruit of Areca catechu	3 liang
三稜	sān léng	Rhizome of Sparganium stoloniferum	3 liang
莪朮	é zhú	Rhizome of Curcumae zedoaria	3 liang
黑醜	hēi chǒu	Seed of Pharbitis nil	3liang
白醜	bái chǒu	Seed of Pharbitis album	3 liang

木香	mù xiāng	Root of Aucklandia lappa	2 liang
甘草	gān cǎo	Root of Glycyrrhiza uralensis	1 liang

Medicinals shall be prepared into water-dewed pills. Dissolve three or four pills in warm water to take in the morning of seizure. Supplement often with warm and thin rice porridge. Not to be taken by expectant mothers, and please abstain from raw food, cold food, buckwheat food, seafood and other fish products.

傷暑

人感此症，必然頭暈、口渴、惡熱。甚則痰多，身熱氣喘。方用：

人參壹錢、白朮伍錢、茯苓三錢、甘草壹錢、青蒿壹兩、香薷三錢、陳皮壹錢。水煎服，一劑愈。

Summer Heat Damage

Patients of *summer heat damage*[13] invariably have symptoms of dizziness, thirst, and *aversion to heat*[14]. The exacerbated cases have profuse phlegm, fever, and panting.

---

[13] *summer heat damage*: a general term for conditions caused by summer heat, especially in mild cases of heatstroke and sunstroke.

[14] *aversion to heat:* strong dislike of heat, also known as heat intolerance.

Formula:

人參	rén shēn	Root of Panax ginseng	1 qian
白朮	bái zhú	Rhizome of Atractylodes macrocephala	5 qian
茯苓	fú líng	Dried fungus of Poria cocos	3 qian
甘草	gān cǎo	Root of Glycyrrhiza uralensis	1 qian
青蒿	qīng hāo	Foliage of Artemisiae Apiacceae	1 liang
香薷	xiāng rú	Herb of Elsholtzia haichowensis	3 qian
陳皮	chén pí	Peel of Citrus reticulata	1 qian

One dose cures.

大滿

此邪在上焦，壅塞而不得散也。方用：

瓜蔞壹個搗碎、枳殼、天花粉各三錢、梔子貳錢、陳皮三錢、厚樸壹錢伍分、半夏、甘草各壹錢，水煎服。

此方之妙，全在用瓜蔞，能去胸膈之食，而消上焦之痰；況又佐以枳殼、花粉，同是消中聖藥；又有厚樸、半夏，以消胃口之痰；尤妙在甘草，使群藥留中而不速下，則邪氣不能久存而散矣。

Serious Indigestion

Serious indigestion is due to pathogens in the *upper energizer*[15], which gives rise to congestion that is not dispersed. Formula:

瓜蔞 guā lóu Fruit of Trichosanthes kirilowii (crumbled) 1pc.

枳殼	zhǐ ké	Dried peel of Aurantii fructus	3 qian
天花粉	tiān huā fěn	Root of Trichosanthes kirilowii	3 qian
梔子	zhī zǐ	Fruit of Gardenia jasminoides	2 qian
陳皮	chén pí	Peel of Citrus reticulata	3 qian
厚樸	hòu pò	Bark of Magnolia officinalis	1.5 qian
半夏	bàn xià	Rhizome of Pinellia ternata	1 qian
甘草	gān cǎo	Root of Glycyrrhiza uralensis	1 qian

The genius of this formula lies in its use of **guā lóu** which removes food retention felt at the chest and eliminates phlegm from the upper energizer. Moreover, **zhǐ ké** and **tiān huā fěn**, two magic medicinals for *resolution*[16] are

---

[15] *upper energizer*: the chest cavity, i.e., the portion above the diaphragm housing the heart and lung, also known as upper burner.

[16] *resolution*: (消中, xiāo zhōng) refers to one of the eight methods of

employed for assistance. **Hòu pǔ** and **bàn xià** resolves *phlegm*[17] at the mouth of stomach. More genius lies in the formula's use of **gān cǎo**, which retains the medicinal efficacy in human body instead of decending rapidly, so that pathogens cannot long survive but disperse.

發汗

凡人邪居腠理之間，必須用汗藥以洩之，方用：

荊芥、防風、甘草、桔梗、蘇葉各壹錢,、白朮伍錢、雲苓三錢、陳皮伍分。水煎服。

此方妙在君白朮，蓋人之脾胃健，而後皮毛腠理始得開合自如，白朮健脾去溼，而邪已難存，況有荊、防、蘇、梗以表散之乎。

Sweat Promotion

Whenever people suffer from pathogens lodged in

treatment: "汗法、吐法、下法、和法、溫法、清法、消法、補法" respectively as "diaphoresis, emesis, purgation, mediation, warming, clearing, resolution and tonification".

17 *phlegm*: phlegm is a complex notion in TCM, it refers to (1) pathologic secretions of the diseased respiratory tract, which is known as sputum; (2) the viscous turbid pathological product that can accumulate in the body, causing a variety of diseases.

their *interstitial*[18] space, medicinals for sweat promotion will be employed for discharging. Formula:

荆芥	jīng jiè	Leaf of Schizonepeta tenuifolia	1 qian
防風	fáng fēng	Root of Ledebouriella divaricata	1 qian
甘草	gān cǎo	Root of Glycyrrhiza uralensis	1 qian
桔梗	jié gěng	Root of Platycodon grandiflorum	1 qian
蘇葉	sū yè	Foliage of Perilla frutescens	1 qian
白朮	bái zhú	Rhizome of Atractylodes macrocephala	5 qian
雲苓	*yún líng*[19]	Dried fungus of Poria cocos	3 qian
陳皮	chén pí	Peel of Citrus reticulata	5 fen

The genius of this formula lies in its use of **bái zhú** as the sovereign herb. If a person's spleen and stomach are healthy, his skin, body hair, and interstices are able to open and close freely in their own rights. **Bái zhú** strengthens spleen and eliminates dampness so that pathogens can hardly

[18] *Interstitial (interstices):* a term referring to the striae of the skin, muscles, and viscera, and also to the tissue between the skin and muscles.

[19] *yún líng: yún líng* refers to the Dried fungus of Poria cocos grown in the southern Yunnan Province of China.

survive, let alone the exterior dissipation of **jīng jiè**, **fáng fēng**, **sū yè** and **jié gěng**.

寒熱真假辨

真熱證：口乾極而呼水，舌燥極而開裂，生刺喉痛，日夜不已，大熱烙手而無汗也；

真寒證：手足寒久而不回，色變青紫，身戰不已，口噤出聲而不可禁也。

假熱證：口雖渴而不甚，舌雖乾而不燥，即燥而無芒、刺紋裂也；

假寒證：手足冰冷，而時有溫和，厥逆身戰亦未太甚，而有時而定，有時而搐是也。

To Differentiate True or False Cold and Heat

True heat disease has symptoms of extremely dry mouth, calling for water, extremely dry and cracked tongue, sharp and achy pain in the throat that lasts day and night, and great heat that burns the hands but with no sweating.

True cold disease has symptoms of chronic cold of the extremities, purple and green-bluish complexion, helpless shivering, clenched jaw, and patient's mouth gives sound involuntarily.

False heat has symptoms of thirst though not severe, patient's tongue is dry but not burning dry, *i.e.* dry but without thorns or cracks.

Symptoms of false cold are ice-cold hands and feet which occasionally become warm, reversal flow, shivering though not extremely. And there is now relief and now convulsion.

乍寒乍熱辨

玩此可知治瘧有用小柴胡湯之法。

病有灑淅惡寒而後發熱者，蓋陰脈不足，陽往從之，陽脈不足，陰往乘之。

何謂陽不足？寸脈微，名曰陽不足，陰氣上入陽中，則惡寒也；何謂陰不足？尺脈弱，名曰陰不足，陽氣下陷陰中，則發熱也。

凡治寒熱，用柴胡升陽氣，使不下陷陰中，則不熱也；用黃芩降陰氣，使不升入陽中，則不寒也。

To Differentiate Sudden Heat and Sudden Cold

By now we know that *Xiao Chai Hu Tang* [pinyin:

xiǎo chái hú tāng, 小柴胡汤, *Minor Bupleurum Decoction*[20]] is one of the therapies for malaria.

Symptoms of patients' aversion to cold, as if having been caught in rain with subsequent fever, is due to deficiency of yin vessels which has been taken advantage by yang , or due to yang vessels deficiency which is exploited by yin.

What is yang deficiency? When speaking of yang deficiency, we think of a deficient *cun*[21] pulse. Yin qi4 ascends and enters into yang to cause aversion to cold. What is yin deficiency? A deficient *chi* pulse is named as yin deficiency. Yang qi4 sinks into yin and cause fever.

For treatment, **chái hú** is employed to *upraise yang qi4*[22], which restrains qi4 from descending into yin and stops

---

[20] *Minor Bupleurum Tang*: Decoction prepared according to *Xiao Chai Hu Formula* (小柴胡方), also known as Minor Bupleurum Formula. It is often used to enhance liver health.

[21] *Cun, guan* and *chi*: the three sections over the radial artery for feeling the pulse: The bar/guan is just central to the radial styloid at the wrist, where the tip of the physician's middle finger is placed, the inch/cun is next to it on the distal side where the tip of the physician's index finger rests, and the cubit/chi is on the proximal side where the tip of the physician's ring finger is placed.

[22] *Upraise yang qi4*: also know as "upraise the middle qi4", it is a

fever; **Huáng qín** is used to downbear yin qi4, which restrains it from ascending and there will not be any cold.

真熱症

方用：

麻黃、黃連、黃芩、石膏、知母、半夏各三錢、當歸伍錢、枳殼貳錢、甘草壹錢。水煎服，一劑輕，二劑愈。

True Heat

Formula:

麻黃	má huáng	Stalk of Ephedra sinica	3 qian
黃連	huáng lián	Rhizome of Coptis chinensis	3 qian
黃芩	huáng qín	Root of Scutellaria baicalensis	3 qian
石膏	shí gāo	Gypsum	3 qian
知母	zhī mǔ	Root of Anemarrhena asphodeloides	3 qian
半夏	bàn xià	Rhizome of Pinellia ternate	3 qian
當歸	dāng guī	Root of Angelica polimorpha	5 qian
枳殼	zhǐ ké	Dried peel of Aurantii fructus	2 qian
甘草	gān cǎo	Root of Glycyrrhiza uralensis	1 qian

therapeutic method to treat sunken middle qi4 by using qi-tonifying medicinals with upraising actions.

The first dose alleviates and the second dose cures.

真寒症

方用：

附子三錢、肉桂、乾薑各壹錢、白朮伍錢、人參壹兩。水煎服，急救之。

此乃真中寒邪，腎火避出軀殼之外，而陰邪之氣，直犯心宮，心君不守，肝氣無依。乃發戰發噤，手足現青色。然則用桂、附、乾薑逐其寒邪足矣，何用參朮？即用何至多加？蓋元陽飛越，祇一線之氣未絕，純用桂、附、乾薑一派辛辣之藥，邪雖外逐，而正氣垂絕。若不多加參朮，何以反正氣於若存若亡之際哉。

True Cold

Formula:

附子	fù zǐ	Lateral root of Aconitum carmichaeli	3 qian
肉桂	ròu guì	Bark of Cinnamonum cassia	1 qian
乾薑	gān jiāng	Dried root of Zingiber officinale	1 qian
白朮	bái zhú	Rhizome of Atractylodes macrocephala	5 qian
人參	rén shēn	Root of Panax ginseng	1 liang

The decoction shall be taken urgently.

True cold is due to contraction of pathogenic cold. Kidney fire escapes to the exteriors of body as yin pathogens attack heart chamber, thus the heart can no longer resist and liver qi4 has nowhere to depend. Patients shiver and are unable to talk; their hands and feet show a green-bluish color. While it is enough to use **fù zǐ**, **ròu guì**, and **gān jiāng** to expel pathogenic cold, why are **rén shēn** and **bái zhú** employed here? And in such a heavy dosage? It is because the *yuan yang* (元陽, primordial yang) has departed leaving a slight trace of qi4 near extinguishing. If only the acrid herbs of **fù zǐ**, **ròu guì**, and **gān jiāng** were used, pathogens would indeed have been expelled, but the upright qi4 might as well have been extinguished. If **bái zhú** and **rén shēn** were not profusely prescribed, the upright qi4 would not be saved at this crucial moment.

假熱症

方用：

黃連、當歸、白芍、半夏各三錢、茯苓、柴胡、梔子各貳錢、枳殼壹錢、菖蒲參分，水煎服。

此方妙在用黃連入心宮，佐以梔子，提刀直入，無邪不散；柴胡、白芍，又塞敵運糧之道；半夏、枳殼，斬殺黨餘。中原既定，四隅不戰而歸。然火勢居中，非用之得法，則賊勢彌張，依然復入。又加菖蒲之辛熱，乘熱飲之，則熱喜熱，不致相反而更相濟也。

False Heat

Formula:

黃連	huáng lián	Rhizome of Coptis chinensis	3 qian
當歸	dāng guī	Root of Angelica polimorpha	3 qian
白芍	bái sháo	Root of Paeonia lactiflora	3 qian
半夏	bàn xià	Rhizome of Pinellia ternata	3 qian
茯苓	fú líng	Dried fungus of Poria cocos	2 qian
柴胡	chái hú	Root of Bupleurum chinense	2 qian
梔子	zhī zǐ	Fruit of Gardenia jasminoides	2 qian
枳殼	zhǐ ké	Dried peel of Aurantii fructus	1 qian
菖蒲	chāng pú	Rhizome of Acorus gramineus	3 fen

The genuis of this formula lies in its combined use of

huáng lián and **zhī zǐ,** medicinal strength of which enters directly into the heart palace and disperses all pathogens. **Chái hú** and **bái sháo** block enemy's flow of supplies, while **bàn xià** and **zhǐ ké** sweep and kill all the remnants. Since the overall situation is stabilized, we can win minor battles with hands down. However, fire exists in the middle and pathogens may rampage if not properly treated. Acrid-hot property of **chāng pú** is strengthened by drinking hot since the high temperature of decoction favors the hot nature of the medicinals, which helps to complement the formula, rather than the contrary.

假寒症

方用：

肉桂、附子各壹錢、人參三錢、白朮伍錢、豬膽汁半個、苦菜汁拾參匙。

水三盃，煎一盃，冷服將藥並器放冷水中，激涼入膽蔡汁調勻，一氣服之。

方中全是熱藥，倘服不如式，必然虛火上沖，將藥嘔出。必熱藥涼服，已足順其性，況下行又有二汁之苦，以騙其假道之防也哉。

False Cold

Formula:

肉桂	ròuguì	Bark of Cinnamonum cassia	1 qian
附子	fù zǐ	Lateral root of Aconitum carmichaeli	1 qian
人參	rén shēn	Root of Panax ginseng	3 qian
白朮	báizhú	Rhizome of Atractylodes macrocephala	5 qian
豬膽汁	zhū dǎn zhī	Bile of Sus scrofa domestica	half piece
苦菜汁	kǔ cài zhī	Juice of Sonchi oleracei	13 spoonfuls

Decoct the medicinals in three cups of water into one cup of docoction, and put the container in cold water to cool. Mix the decoction well with **zhū dǎn zhī** and **kǔ cài zhī**, and drink it at one draft.

All medicinals employed are of hot propterty in nature. If not prepared in this way, deficiency fire would flame upward and patients would vomit upon taking the decoction. That hot medicinals shall be drunk cold is a respect to their natural property. With the company of bitter medicinals of **kǔ cài zhī** and **zhū dǎn zhī**, hot-property medicinals take effect by way of the cold-natured ones. What a deception on the enemy!

真熱假寒

此症身外冰冷，身内火熾，發寒發熱，戰慄不已，乃真熱反現假寒之象以欺人也。

法當用三黄湯加石膏生薑，乘熱飲之，再用井水以撲其心，至二三十次，内熱自止，外之戰慄亦若失矣。

後用元參、麥冬、白芍各二兩煎湯，任其恣飲，後不再甚也。

True Heat with False Cold

The symptoms of *true heat with false cold*[23] include ice-cold exterior with intense internal fever, alternating cold and fever, and helpless shivering and trembling. The true heat can be in disguise of false cold.

The prescription is *San Huang Tan*g [pinyin: sān huáng tāng, 三黄湯, Three Huang Decoction] prepared with **shí gāo** and **shēng jiāng**. Drink hot and then use well water to cool the patient's chest. In twenty or thirty times, the internal heat ceases and the external shivering dwindles away.

---

23 *true heat with false cold*: a pathological change marked by excessive heat in the interior with pseudo-cold manifestations.

After this treatment, prepare a decoction of two *liang* of **yuán shēn**, **mài dōng**, and **bái sháo** respectively for drinking in free dosage. It prevents any possible deterioration.

真寒假熱

此症下部冰冷，上部大熱，渴欲飲水，下喉即吐，乃真寒反現假熱之形以欺人也。

法當用八味湯，大劑探冷與服，再令人以手擦其足心，如火之熱，不熱不已，以大熱為度。

用吳萸一兩，附子一錢，麝香三分，以少許白麵入之，打糊作膏，貼足心，少頃必睡，醒來下部熱，而上之火息矣。

True Cold with False Heat

The symptom of true cold with false heat is coldness in lower body with great heat in the upper. Patient is thirsty with a strong desire to drink water but may vomit upon drinking. True cold can appear with deceptive symptoms of false heat.

The prescription is a large dose of *Ba Wei Tang*[24] [pinyin: bā wèi tāng, 八味湯, Eight-medicinal Decoction] to be taken cold, and then rub patient's soles vigorously till they are burning hot.

Flour batter is prepared with one liang of **wú yú**, one qian of **fù zǐ**, three fen of **shè xiāng** and a certain amount of wheat flour. Paste the prepared plaster to the soles of patient who will fall asleep soon. When he wakes up, his lower body is warmed and the upper fire is extinguished.

上熱下寒

此症上焦火盛，吐痰如湧泉，面赤喉痛，上身不欲蓋衣，而下身冰冷，此上假熱而下真寒也，方用：

附子壹個、熟地半斤、山萸肆兩、麥冬壹兩、茯苓三兩、伍味子壹兩、丹皮參兩、澤瀉參兩、肉桂壹兩。

水十碗，煎三碗，探冷與服，其渣再用水三碗，煎一碗，一氣服之，立刻安靜，此上病下治之法也。

---

24 *Ba Wei Tang:* Eight-medicinal Decoction, 八味湯, Source of formula: Vol.4, *Yi Che* (醫徹).

Upper Body Heat and Lower Body Cold

The symptoms of *upper body heat and lower body cold*[25] are scorching fire in the upper energizer, phlegm that bubbles up like a spring, flushed complexion and a sore throat. The upper body desires nakedness, and the lower body is ice-cold. This is false heat of the upper body and true cold of the lower. Formula:

附子 fù zǐ Lateral root of Aconitum carmichaeli 1 piece
熟地 shú dì Prepared root of Rehmannia glutinosa half *jin*[26]
山萸 shān yú Fruit of Cornus officinalis 4 liang
麥冬 mài dōng Tuber of Ophiopogon japonicus 1 liang
茯苓 fú líng Dried fungus of Poria cocos 3 liang
伍味子 wǔ wèi zǐ Fruit of Schisandra chinensis 1 liang
丹皮 dān pí Bark of the root of Paeonia suffruticosa 3 liang
澤瀉 zé xiè Rhizome of Alisma plantago-aquatica 3 liang
肉桂 ròu guì Bark of Cinnamonum cassia 1 liang

---

[25] *upper body heat and lower body cold* is a complex condition characterized by simultaneous presence of heat in the upper body and cold in the lower, the same as heat above and cold below.

[26] *jin:* a weight unit of China, one *jin* equals half of a kilo.

Decoct the medicinals in ten bowls of water down to three bowls and drink the decoction cold. Then, three bowls of water with the dregs are decocted into one bowl for drinking at one draft. Then, patient calms down immediately. This is a way that upper body disease is treated through the lower[27].

循衣撮空

此症非大實則大虛，當審其因，察其脈，參其症而分黑白矣，實而便秘者，大承氣湯，虛而便滑者，獨參湯，厥逆者加附子。

Carphology and Floccilation

Carphology and floccilation[28] is due either to extreme excess or to extreme deficiency. Symptoms should be carefully differentiated through studying the causes and inspecting the pulses. For excess with constipation, we

---

[27] Considering the large quantity of each medicinal, this formula is probably for 10 doses of decoction instead of one dose only.

[28] *Carphology*: Picking at the bedclothes, a sign of death. *Floccilation*: Groping in the air, a sign of death.

should use *Da Cheng Qi4 Tang*[29] [pinyin: dà chéng qì tāng, 大承氣湯, Major Drastic Purgative Decoction]. In case of deficiency with slippery stools, prescribe *Du Shen Tang* [pinyin: dú shēn tāng, 獨參湯, Single Ginseng Decoction]. In case of reversal cold, add **fù zǐ** in it.

陰虛雙蛾

方用：

附子壹錢，鹽水炒，每用一片含口中，後以六味地黃湯，大劑飲之。附外治法：

引火下行，用附子一個為末，醋調貼湧泉穴，或吳萸一兩，白麵伍錢水調貼湧泉穴，急針刺少商穴，則咽喉有一線之路矣。

Tonsillitis Due to Yin Deficiency

Formula:

One qian of **fù zǐ** sautéed in salt water. Let patient take one piece of **fù zǐ** in mouth, and then drink a large dose of

---

29 *Da Cheng Qi4 Tang* (大承氣湯), formula:大黃 dài huáng (12g),厚樸 hòu pò (15g), 枳實 zhǐshí (12g), 芒硝 máng xiāo (9g). Source of formula: On Cold Damage(傷寒論).

Liu Wei Di Huang Tang[30] [pinyin: liù wèi dì huáng tāng, 六味地黃湯, Decoction of Six Ingredients with Rehmannia]. An external therapy is also attached:

Conduct fire[31] downward by mixing powdered **fù zǐ** (one piece) with vinegar, and plaster the mixture to patient's Yongquan point LU11. Alternatively, mix one liang of **wú yú** with five qian of wheat flour and water, and plaster the mixture to Yongquan point LU11, and then instantly needle Shaoshang point KI1, which may relieve the symptom by opening up a narrow way in the patient's throat.

結胸

此傷寒之變症也，傷寒邪火正熾，不可急於飲食，飲

---

[30] *Liu Wei Di Huang Tang*: Liu Wei Di Huang Decoction, also used as *Liuwei Dihuang teapills* (六味地黃丸: liù wèi dì huáng wán), is a famous prescription in TCM and pharmacy. The formula was created by Qian Yi (錢乙: Qián Yǐ) as Dihuang pill (地黃丸). It was published in "Xiao'er Yao Zheng Zhi Jue" ("Key to Therapeutics of Children's Diseases", 小兒藥證直訣: Xiǎo'ér Yào Zhèng Zhí Jué) in 1119 by Qian Yi's student.

[31] *conduct fire (back to its origin)*: a therapeutic principle for the ascending of asthenic fire, by adding drugs for tonifying the kidney yang to those for nourishing the kidney yin to lead the ascending deficiency fire back down to the kidney, the same as to conduct fire downward.

食而成此者。方用：瓜蔞壹個搥碎，甘草壹錢。水煎服，勿遲。

瓜蔞乃結胸之聖藥，常人服之，必至心如遺若，病人服之，不畏其虛乎，不知結胸之症，是食在胸中，非大黃、枳殼、檳榔、厚樸所能祛逐，必得瓜蔞，始得推蕩鬭脾，少加甘草以和之，不致十分猛烈也。

Chest Bind

Chest bind[32] is a transformed symptom of cold damage. When the pathogenic fire of cold damage blazes, patient's diet should be halted, otherwise chest bind forms. Formula:

One piece of **guā lóu** is crumbled and decocted with one qian of **gān cǎo** for intake without delay.

Guā lóu, a magic medicinal for chest bind, brings about a feeling of chest emptiness even if taken by healthy people. Should not patients fear deficiency if they take **guā lóu**? Those asking this question ignore a fact that chest bind is the result of congested food and can in no way be removed by medicinals like **dà huáng**, **zhǐ ké**, **bīng láng** and **hòu pò**.

[32] *Chest bind*: a diseased state attributable to accumulation of pathogens in the chest and abdomen, often manifested by local rigidity, fullness and tenderness, also named as chest constriction.

Only by adding **guā lóu**, can they push away the blockage and open up spleen. Moreover, a small amount of **gān cǎo** should also be prescriped to moderate its ferocious efficacy.

扶正散邪湯

人參、半夏、甘草各壹錢、白朮、茯苓、柴胡各三錢。水煎服。

此方專治正氣虛而邪氣入之者，如頭痛發熱，右寸脈大於左寸口者，急以此方投之，無不全愈。

Decoction for Supporting Right Qi4 and Dissipating Pathogens

人參	rén shēn	Root of Panax ginseng	1 qian
半夏	bàn xià	Rhizome of Pinellia ternata	1 qian
甘草	gān cǎo	Root of Glycyrrhiza uralensis	1 qian
白朮	bái zhú	Rhizome of Atractylodes macrocephala	3 qian
茯苓	fú líng	Dried fungus of Poria cocos	3 qian
柴胡	chái hú	Root of Bupleurum chinense	3 qian

This is a specialized formula for treating upright qi4 deficiency under invasion of pathogenic qi4. The symptoms are headache, fever, and that the right cun pulse is felt stronger than the left cun pulse. Instant prescription of this formula cures with no exception.

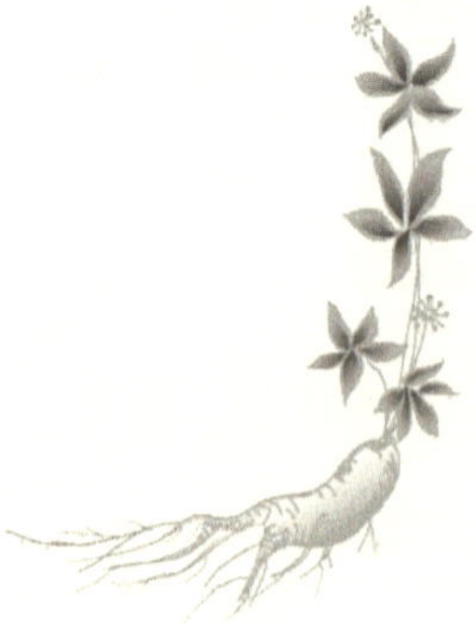

火證門

Chapter 2　Fire Syndrome

瀉火湯總方

梔子、丹皮各叁錢，白芍五錢，元參貳錢，甘草壹錢，水煎服。

心火加黃連一錢，胃火加生石膏三錢，腎火加黃柏、知母各一錢，肺火加黃芩一錢，大腸火加地榆一錢，小腸火加天冬、麥冬各一錢，膀胱火加澤瀉三錢。

治火何獨治肝經？蓋肝屬木，最易生火。肝火散，則諸經之火俱散。但散火必須用下洩之藥，而使火之有出路也則得矣。

Fire-purging[33] Decoction - A General Formula

梔子	zhī zǐ	Fruit of Gardenia jasminoides	3 qian
丹皮	dān pí	Bark of the root of Paeonia suffruticosa	3 qian
白芍	bái sháo	Root of Paeonia lactiflora	5 qian
元參	*yuán shēn*[34]	Root of Scrophularia ningpoensis	2 qian

---

[33] *purge fire*: a therapeutic method of removing pathogenic fire by using bitter-cold medicinals.

甘草 gān cǎo Root of Glycyrrhiza uralensis 1 qian

For heart fire, add one qian of **huáng lián**; For stomach fire, add three qian of **shēng shí gāo**; For kidney fire, add one qian of **huáng bǎi** and **zhī mǔ** respectively; For lung fire, add one qian of **huáng qín**; For *large intestine*[35] fire, add one qian of **dì yú**; For *small intestine*[36] fire, add one qian of **tiān dōng** and **mài dōng** respectively; For bladder fire, add three qian of **zé xiè**.

Why is the liver meridian purged of fire in this formula only? It is because liver corresponds to wood and is the easiest place to catch fire. Once *liver fire*[37] is dispersed, all fire of other meridians will extinguish. But in order to do that, purgative medicinals must be applied so that the fire may have an exit to go.

---

34 *yuán shēn*: 元参, an alternate name for 玄参.

35 *large intestine*: one of the six bowels, it receives waste from the small intestine and then forms it into stool before discharging.

36 *small intestine*: one of the six bowels, whose main function is to receive food content of the stomach, further digest it and absorb nutrients and water.

37 *liver fire*: a pathological change of exuberant liver qi4 with heat manifestations.

火證

真火證，初起必大渴引飲，身有斑點，或身熱如焚，或發狂亂語。方用：

石膏、知母、升麻、半夏、甘草各叁錢，元參、麥冬各壹兩，竹葉壹伯片，水煎服。一劑少止，三劑愈。

大寒之證亦有發斑者，但看其渴與不渴。若身發斑不渴、小飲即吐飲，雖沸湯不覺甚熱，此大寒證，不可與此。

Fire Syndrome

The true fire syndrome invariably begins with patient's extreme thirst for water, speckled skin, madness, gibberish and possibly a burning-hot body. Formula:

石膏	shí gāo	Gypsum	3 qian
知母	zhī mǔ	Root of Anemarrhena asphodeloides	3 qian
升麻	shēng má	Rhizome of Cimifuga foetida	3 qian
半夏	bàn xià	Rhizome of Pinellia ternate	3 qian
甘草	gān cǎo	Root of Glycyrrhiza uralensis	3 qian
元參	yuán shēn	Root of Scrophularia ningpoensis	1 liang
麥冬	mài dōng	Tuber of Ophiopogon japonicus	1 liang
竹葉	zhú yè	Foliage of Phyllostachys	100 pcs.

The first dose alleviates and the third dose cures.

Great cold syndrome might as well be symptomized by speckled skin. The thirst is the decisive factor in here. If patient has a speckled body without thirst, vomits upon drinking even a small amount, and does not feel hot even when drinking boiling-hot water, he must have great cold syndrome, and this formula is not applicable.

火越

此乃胃火與肝火共騰而外越，不為丹毒，即為痧疹，非他火也。方用：

元參壹兩，乾葛參兩，升麻、青蒿、黃耆各叁錢，水煎服。

此方妙在用青蒿，肝胃之火俱平，又佐以群藥重劑，而火安有不滅者乎？治小兒亦效。

Fire Overflow

This is due to the joint rising of both stomach fire and liver fire, which results in either *erysipelas*[38] or *exanthum*[39].

[38] *erysipelas*: an acute infection of the skin marked by intense local redness.

[39] *exanthum*: a general term for skin eruption or rash, but usually

Formula:

元參	yuán shēn	Root of Scrophularia ningpoensis	1 liang
乾葛	gān gē	Root of Pueraria lobata	3 liang
升麻	shēng má	Rhizome of Cimifuga foetida	3 qian
青蒿	qīng hāo	Foliage of Artemisiae Apiacceae	3 qian
黃耆	huáng qí	Root of Astragalus membranaceus	3 qian

Genius of this formula lies in its use of **qīng hāo**, which normalizes both liver and stomach fire. Meanwhile, other medicinals in heavy doses are also applied for assistance. How can the fire stay? The formula is also applicable to children.

燥證

此證初起，喉乾口渴，乾燥不吐痰，乾咳嗽不已，面色日紅，不畏風吹者是也。方用：

麥冬、元參各伍錢，桔梗叁錢，花粉、甘草各壹錢，陳皮參分，百部捌分，水煎服。

---

referring to measles.

Dryness[40] Syndrome

On onset, dryness syndrome has symptoms of dry throat, thirst, *dry retching*[41] without expectoration. There is also dry and helpless cough, and patient's complexion is reddened day by day while with no aversion to wind. Formula:

麥冬	mài dōng	Tuber of Ophiopogon japonicus	5 qian
元參	yuán shēn	Root of Scrophularia ningpoensis	5 qian
桔梗	jié gěng	Root of Platycodon grandiflorum	3 qian
花粉	huā fěn	Seed of Trichosanthes kirilowii	1 qian
甘草	gān cǎo	Root of Glycyrrhiza uralensis	1 qian
陳皮	chén pí	Peel of Citrus reticulata	3 fen
百部	bǎi bù	Root of Sessile Stemona	8 fen

治火丹神方

絲瓜子、元參各壹兩，柴胡、升麻各壹錢，當歸伍錢，

[40] *dryness*: dryness as a pathogenic factor characterized by dryness and is apt to injure the lung and consume fluid, also called pathogenic dryness.

[41] *dry retching:* a noisy involuntary effort to vomit, but without bringing anything up from the stomach.

水煎服。小兒服之亦效。

A Magic Formula for *Erysipelas*

絲瓜子	sī guā zǐ	Seed of Luffa cylindrica(L.) Roem.	1 liang
元參	yuán shēn	Root of Scrophularia ningpoensis	1 liang
柴胡	chái hú	Root of Bupleurum chinense	1 qian
升麻	shēng má	Rhizome of Cimifuga foetida	1 qian
當歸	dāng guī	Root of Angelica polimorpha	5 qian

It is also effective if applied to children.

消食病

此火盛之證，大渴引飲，呼水自救，朝食即飢，或夜食不止。方用：

元參壹兩，麥冬伍錢，生地叁錢，竹葉參拾片，菊花、白芥子、丹皮各貳錢，陳皮伍分，水煎服。

Excess Hunger

As a result of excessive fire, excess hunger is symptomized by patient’s great thirst and crying out for water. Patients feel hunger even just after food intake in the day, and may eat incessantly at night. Formula:

元參	yuán shēn	Root of Scrophularia ningpoensis	1 liang
麥冬	mài dōng	Tuber of Ophiopogon japonicus	5 qian
生地	shēng dì	Fresh root of Rehmannia glutinosa	3 qian
竹葉	zhú yè	Foliage of Phyllostachys	30 pieces
菊花	jú huā	Flower of Chrysanthemum morafolii	2 qian
白芥子	bái jiè zǐ	Seed of Brassica alba	2 qian
丹皮	dān pí	Bark of the root of Paeonia suffruticosa	2 qian
陳皮	chén pí	Peel of Citrus reticulata	5 fen

痿證

不能起床，已成廢人者，此乃火盛內熾，腎水熬乾。治法宜降胃火而補腎水。方用降補湯：

熟地、元參、麥冬各壹兩，甘菊花、生地、沙參、地骨皮各伍錢，車前子貳錢，人參叁錢，水煎服。

Wilting[42] Syndrome

Sufferers are unable to rise to his feet and are totally handicapped. This is due to excessive fire blazing internally, which simmers dry their kidney water. It is a proper

---

42 *wilting*: weakness and limpness of the sinews that in severe cases leads to muscular atrophy and prevents the lifting of the legs and arms, the same as atrophy-flaccidity.

treatment to reduce stomach fire with supplementing kidney water. Formula: *Jiang Bu Tang* [pinyin: jiàng bǔ tāng, 降補湯, Downbearing and Supplementation Decoction]

熟地 shú dì Prepared root of Rehmannia glutinosa 1 liang
元參 yuán shēn Root of Scrophularia ningpoensis 1 liang
麥冬 mài dōng Tuber of Ophiopogon japonicus 1 liang
甘菊花 *gān jú huā*[43] Flowers of Chrysanthemum morafolii 5 qian
生地 shēng dì Fresh root of Rehmannia glutinosa 5 qian
沙參 shā shēn Root of Adenophora tetraphylla 5 qian
地骨皮 dì gǔ pí Bark of the root of Lycium chinensis 5 qian
車前子 chē qián zǐ Seed of Plantago asiatica 2 qian
人參 rén shēn Root of Panax ginseng 3 qian

痿證

人有兩足無力，不能起立，而口又健飯，少飢則頭面皆熱，咳嗽不已，此亦痿證。方用起痿至神湯：

熟地、元參、山藥、菊花各壹兩，當歸、白芍、人參各伍錢，神麯貳錢，白芥子叁錢，水煎服。三十劑而愈。

---

[43] *gān jú huā* is 菊花(jú huā) that comes from Canton.

Wilting Syndrome

Patients lack strength in their feet, cannot rise and are food addicted. Their head and face are hot and they cough helplessly even if with slight hunger. These are also symptoms of wilting syndrome. Formula: *Qi Wei Zhi Shen Tang* [pinyin: qǐ wěi zhì shén tāng, 起痿至神湯, Sovereign Remedy for Removing Wilt]

熟地	shú dì	Prepared root of Rehmannia glutinosa	1 liang
元參	yuán shēn	Root of Scrophularia ningpoensis	1 liang
山藥	shān yào	Root of Dioscorea opposita	1 liang
菊花	jú huā	Flower of Chrysanthemum morafolii	1 liang
當歸	dāng guī	Root of Angelica polimorpha	5 qian
白芍	bái sháo	Root of Paeonia lactiflora	5 qian
人參	rén shēn	Root of Panax ginseng	5 qian
神麴	shén qū	Medicated leaven	2 qian
白芥子	bái jiè zǐ	Seed of Brassica alba	3 qian

It is cured in thirty doses.

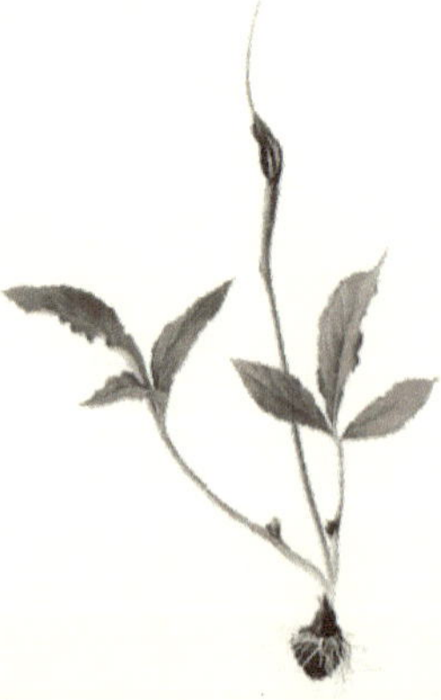

郁結門

Chapter 3 Depressive Stagnation

開鬱

如人頭痛身熱，傷風咳嗽，或心不爽，而鬱氣蘊於中懷，或氣不舒，而怒氣留於脅下，斷不可用補藥。方用：

當歸叁錢、白芍伍錢、半夏貳錢、枳殼、薄荷、白朮、丹皮、甘草各壹錢，水煎服。

頭痛加川芎一錢，目痛加蒺藜一錢，菊花一錢，鼻塞加蘇葉一錢，喉痛加桔梗二錢，肩背痛加枳殼羌活，兩手痛加薑黃或桂枝一錢。腹痛不可按者，加大黃二錢，按之而不痛者，加肉桂(壹錢)，餘不必加。

Depression Relief

Symptoms like headache, fever, wind damage, cough, and a bad mood of patient, may result in embedded qi4 of depression and constraint of qi4, which may further lead to angery qi4 stagnated at the body sides of patient. For these symptoms, the tonifying medicinals should be strictly prohibited. Formula:

當歸	dāng guī	Root of Angelica polimorpha	3 qian
白芍	bái sháo	Root of Paeonia lactiflora	5 qian
半夏	bàn xià	Rhizome of Pinellia ternata	2 qian
枳殼	zhǐ ké	Dried peel of Aurantii fructus	1 qian
薄荷	bò hé	Plant of Mentha Haplocalyx	1 qian
白朮	bái zhú	Rhizome of Atractylodes macrocephala	1 qian
丹皮	dān pí	Bark of the root of Paeonia suffruticosa	1 qian
甘草	gān cǎo	Root of Glycyrrhiza uralensis	1 qian

For headache, add additional one qian of **chuān xiōng**; For eye pain, add one qian of **jí lí** and **jú huā** respectively; For nasal congestion, add one qian of **sū yè**; For sore throat, add two qian of **jié gěng**; For shoulder and back pain, add **zhǐ ké** and **qiāng huó**. For pain of both hands, add one qian of **jiāng huáng** or one qian of **guì zhī**; For abdominal pain with aversion to pressure, add two qian of **dà huáng.** If the abdominal pain relieves with pressure, then add one qian of **ròu guì.** Other symptoms do not call for any addition of medicinals.

關格

怒氣傷肝，而肝氣沖於胃口之間，腎氣不得上行，肺氣不得下行，而成此證，以開鬱為主，方用：

荊芥、柴胡、川鬱金、茯苓、蘇子、白芥子、花粉各壹錢、白芍叁錢、甘草伍分，水煎服。

又方用：

陰陽水各一碗，加鹽一撮，打百餘下，起泡，飲之即吐而愈。凡上焦有疾，欲吐而不能吐者，飲之立吐。

Block and Repulsion

Anger damages liver, and liver qi4 may surge to stay between stomach and mouth, which restrains the ascending of kidney qi4 and the decending of lung qi4. *Block and repulsion*[44] is thus formed. This formula aims at the removal of stagnation:

荊芥 jīng jiè	Leaf of Schizonepeta tenuifolia	1 qian
柴胡 chái hú	Root of Bupleurum chinense	1 qian
川鬱金 *chuān yù jīn*[45]	Root of Curcuma aromatica	1 qian

44 *block and repulsion*: a diseased state characterized by urinary stoppage and vomit.

45 *chuān yù jīn*: Root of Curcuma aromatica grown in Sichuan Province

茯苓 fú líng	Dried fungus of Poria cocos	1 qian
蘇子 sū zǐ	Seed of Perilla frutescens	1 qian
白芥子 bái jiè zǐ	Seed of Brassica alba	1 qian
花粉 huā fěn	Seed of Trichosanthes kirilowii	1 qian
白芍 bái sháo	Root of Paeonia lactiflora	3 qian
甘草 gān cǎo	Root of Glycyrrhiza uralensis	5 fen

Another formula:

Mix one bowl of yin water and one bowl of yang water (*i.e.* to mix boiled and unboiled water), add a pinch of salt into the mixed water, and swirl the mixture till it bubbles. Patient may vomit upon drinking the solution and the disease is cured. This formula may be applied to any syndrome of the upper energizer to promote vomiting, when patient wants to vomit but unable to.

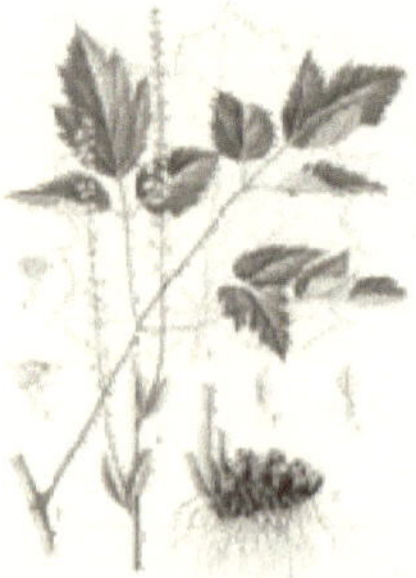

of China.

虛勞門

Chapter 4 Consumptive Disease

癆證虛損辨

二證外相似而治法不同。虛損者，陰陽兩虛也；勞證者，陰虛陽亢也。故虛損可用溫補，若勞證則忌溫補而用清補也。

兩證辨法不必憑脈，但看人著複衣，此著單衣者為勞證；人著單衣，此著複衣者為虛損。勞證骨蒸而熱，虛損營衛虛而熱也。

To Differentiate Exhaustion Syndrome and Deficient Detriment

The two syndromes resemble each other seemingly though they are treated in different ways. Deficient detriment is due to both yin and yang deficiency, while exhaustion syndrome is due to *yin deficiency with yang hyperactivity*[46]. Therefore, *warm tonification*[47] is prescribed

[46] *yin deficiency with yang hyperactivity*: insufficient essence, blood, and fluid failing to restrain yang, causing increased activity of yang.

[47] *warm tonification*: a therapeutic method to treat deficiency-cold

for deficient detriment, and exhaustion syndrome shall be treated with clear supplementation but refrained from warm tonification.

There is no need to take pulse in order to differentiate the two syndromes. It is enough only to look at their clothes. If a patient is clad in a thin coat while healthy people are in heavy garments, the patient must be suffering from exhaustion syndrome. If, on the other hand, the patient wears heavy coat while others in thin clothes, then he is suffering from deficient detriment. For exhaustion syndrome, fever is due to *steaming bone*[48]; whereas for deficient detriment, fever is caused by ying and defensive qi4 deficiency.

內傷發熱

方用：

當歸、柴胡、陳皮、梔子、甘草各壹錢、白芍、花粉各貳錢，水煎服。

凡肝木鬱者，此方一劑即快。人病發熱，有內傷外感，必先散其邪氣，邪退而後補正，則正不為邪所傷也。但外

---

conditions by using warm-tonifying medicinals.

[48] *steam bone:* a subjective feeling of fever deep in the body, which appears to emanate from the bone or marrow.

感內傷，不可用一方也，外感發熱方見前。

Fever of Internal Damage

Formula:

當歸	dāng guī	Root of Angelica polimorpha	1 qian
柴胡	chái hú	Root of Bupleurum chinense	1 qian
陳皮	chén pí	Peel of Citrus reticulata	1 qian
梔子	zhī zǐ	Fruit of Gardenia jasminoides	1 qian
甘草	gān cǎo	Root of Glycyrrhiza uralensis	1 qian
白芍	bái sháo	Root of Paeonia lactiflora	2 qian
花粉	huā fěn	Seed of Trichosanthes kirilowii	2 qian

The formula quickly relieves liver stagnation in a single dose. As for fever of internal damage with external contraction, pathogens must be dispersed firstly, and the right qi4 is tonified after the pathogens' retreat, so that the right qi4 cannot be harmed by the pathogens. It's quite another case for fever of external contraction with internal damage. Please refer to the aforesaid formula for fever of external contraction.

未成勞而將成勞

方用：

熟地壹兩、地骨皮、人三、麥冬各伍錢、白芥子、山藥各三錢、白術壹錢、五味子三分，水煎服。

凡人右寸脈大於左寸即內傷之證，不論左右關尺脈何如，以此方投之效驗。

Pre-consumptive Symptoms

Formula:

熟地 shú dì Prepared root of Rehmannia glutinosa1 liang
地骨皮 dì gŭ pí Bark of the root of Lycium chinensis5 qian
人三 rén sān Root of Panax ginseng 5 qian
麥冬 mài dōng Tuber of Ophiopogon japonicus 5 qian
白芥子 bái jiè zĭ Seed of Brassica alba 3 qian
山藥 shān yào Root of Dioscorea opposita 3 qian
白術 bái zhú Rhizome of Atractylodes macrocephala 1 qian
五味子 wŭ wèi zĭ Fruit of Schisandra chinensis 3 fen

If a patient's right cun pulse is felt stronger than his left cun pulse, it is a syndrome of internal damage. Regardless of what the left or the right guan-chi pulse is, the formula is effective when applied.

陽虛下陷

凡人饑飽勞役，內傷正氣，以致氣乃下行，脾胃不能克化，飲食不能運動，往往變為勞瘵，蓋疑飲食不進為脾胃之病，肉黍之積，輕則砂仁、枳殼、山查、麥芽之品，重則芒硝、大黃、牽牛、巴豆之類，紛然雜進，必致臟悶而漸成勞矣。若先以升提之藥治之，何至於成勞？方用：

人三、柴胡、陳皮、甘草各壹錢、升麻三分、黃耆、白術各三錢。水煎服。

Sunken Yang Deficiency

Irregularity of food intake and hard labor may hurt healthy qi4 internally, which leads to the sinking of healthy qi4 and in turn causes malfunction of spleen and stomach in the process of food movement. The above situations often induce exhaustive consumption, which may be mistaken for a food stagnation disease of the spleen and stomach and treated with **shā rén**, **zhǐ ké**, **shān zhā,** and **mài yá**, or even with **máng xiāo**, **dà huáng**, **qiān niú** and **bā dòu** for exacerbated cases. These assorted medicinals will cause distension of the abdomen which gradually develops into consumptive disease. If treated with upraising medicinals from the very beginning, the consumptive disease would not have resulted. Formula:

人三	rén sān	Root of Panax ginseng	1 qian
柴胡	chái hú	Root of Bupleurum chinense	1 qian
陳皮	chén pí	Peel of Citrus reticulata	1 qian
甘草	gān cǎo	Root of Glycyrrhiza uralensis	1 qian
升麻	shēng má	Rhizome of Cimifuga foetida	3 fen
黄耆	huáng qí	Root of Astragalus membranaceus	3 qian
白術	bái zhú	Rhizome of Atractylodes macrocephala	3 qian

陰虛下陷

凡人陰虛脾洩，歲久不止，或食而不化，或化而溏洩。方用：

熟地壹兩、山藥、山萸、白朮各伍錢、茯苓叁錢、升麻參分、肉桂、五味子、車前子各壹錢。水煎晚服。

此方純是補陰之藥，且有升麻以提陰中之氣，又有溫溼之品以煖命門而健脾土，何至溏洩哉？此證每至，腿腳發踵，稍多飲食即便蛔蟲，乃脾陰虛陷已極，方宜加入乾薑、烏梅。

Yin Deficiency Collapse

A yin-deficient patient who has chronic spleen diarrhea, indigestion, or *sloppy diarrhea*[49] shall be treated with decoction of this formula taken in evening:

熟地	shú dì	Prepared root of Rehmannia glutinosa	1 liang
山藥	shān yào	Root of Dioscorea opposite	5 qian
山萸	shān yú	Fruit of Cornus officinalis	5 qian
白朮	bái zhú	Rhizome of Atractylodes macrocephala	5 qian
茯苓	fú líng	Dried fungus of Poria cocos	3 qian
升麻	shēng má	Rhizome of Cimifuga foetida	3 fen
肉桂	ròu guì	Bark of Cinnamonum cassia	1 qian
五味子	wǔ wèi zǐ	Fruit of Schisandra chinensis	1 qian
車前子	chē qián zǐ	Seed of Plantago asiatica	1 qian

This formula is purely of yin tonification. It uses **shēng má** to upraise qi4 of yin and medidinals warm and wet in

[49] *sloppy diarrhea*: diarrhea with soft, unformed stool.

nature are used to warm the *life gate*[50] and to fortify spleen earth. Then how could there be any sloppy diarrhea? Whenever the syndrome strikes, the patient's legs and feet swell, slightly enlarged diet may lead to feces containing ascaris. This is a symptom of utmost yin deficiency of spleen. It's appropriate to add **gān jiāng** and **wū méi** to the formula.

陰虛火動,夜熱晝寒

此腎水虛兼感寒，或腎水虧竭，夜熱晝寒。若認作陽證治之，則口渴而熱益熾，必致消盡陰水，吐痰如絮，咳嗽不已，聲啞聲嘶，變成勞瘵。法當峻補其陰，而陰水足而火焰消，骨髓清泰矣。方用：

熟地、元三各壹兩，山萸、地骨皮、芡實各伍錢，五味子，麥冬、沙三、白芥子各三錢，桑葉拾肆片，水煎服。

此方治陰虛火動者神效。

Fire Agitation of Yin Deficiency with Fever at Night and Cold in Day

This is the result of concurrent kidney water deficiency

[50] *life gate*: (1) the place where qi4 transformation of the human body originates, serving as the root of life; (2) right kidney; (3) acupuncture point (GV4).

and cold contraction, or of the exhaustion of kidney water with symtoms of fever at night and cold in day. If treated as a yang syndrome, the patient will have symptoms of thirst and a blazing fever that will in turn exhaust yin water. There will also be expectoration of fleecy phlegm, helpless cough and a hoarse voice, which will finally develop into exhaustive consumption. It is a proper treatment to drastically supplement the yin, so that yin water suffices and fire dwindles away, and bone marrow is clear and safe. Formula:

熟地	shú dì	Prepared root of Rehmannia glutinosa	1 liang
元三	yuán sān	Root of Scrophularia ningpoensis	1 liang
山萸	shān yú	Fruit of Cornus officinalis	5 qian
地骨皮	dì gŭ pí	Bark of the root of Lycium chinensis	5 qian
芡實	qiàn shí□	Seed of Gordon Euryale	5 qian
五味子	wŭ wèi zĭ	Fruit of Schisandra chinensis	3 qian
麥冬	mài dōng	Tuber of Ophiopogon japonicus	3 qian
沙三	*shā sān*[51]	Root of Adenophora tetraphylla	3 qian
白芥子	bái jiè zĭ	Seed of Brassica alba	3 qian

[51] *沙三*: shā sān is an alternative name for 沙參 shā shēn.

桑葉 sāng yè Foliage of Mori 40 pcs.

This formula has magic effect in treating fire agitation of yin deficiency.

陰寒無火

方用：

肉桂、柴胡各壹錢，熟地壹兩，附子、白術、人三各三錢，水煎服。

二方治陰之中，即有以治陽；治陽之中，即藏於補陰。此兩方似六味八味地黃，而上方之白芥、桑葉，下方之柴胡，其妙用有過於地黃丸之丹澤者，用者不可以意加減也。

Yin Cold without Fire

Formula:

肉桂	ròu guì	Bark of Cinnamonum cassia	1 qian
柴胡	chái hú	Root of Bupleurum chinense	1 qian
熟地	shú dì	Prepared root of Rehmannia glutinosa	1 liang
附子	fù zǐ	Lateral root of Aconitum carmichaeli	3 qian
白術	bái zhú	Rhizome of Atractylodes macrocephala	3 qian
人三	rén sān	Root of Panax ginseng	3 qian

In the aforsaid two formulae, yin is treated by treating yang, and yin tonification lies in yang treatment. The relationship between these two formulae is similar to that of *Liu Wei Di Huang* and *Ba Wei Di Huang*. **Bái jiè** and **sāng yè** of the former formula and **chái hú** of the latter are used more ingeniously than **mǔ dān pí** and **zé xiè** of *Di Huang Wan*. Proportions of the medicinals should not be adjusted at discretion.

過勞

凡人過勞，脈必浮大不倫，若不安閒作息，必有吐血之證，法當滋補。方用：

熟地、黄芪、白芍、白術各伍兩，山萸肆兩，人三、茯苓、五味子、麥冬□各三兩，神曲壹兩，砂仁、陳皮各五錢，當歸半斤。

蜜丸，早晚滾開水送下五錢。

Overwork

Patients of overwork invariably have extremely floating and abnormal pulses. If not to rest properly, they will have blood ejection syndrome. The prescription is to enrich and supplement. Formula:

熟地	shú dì	Prepared root of Rehmannia glutinosa	5 liang
黃耆	huáng qí	Root of Astragalus membranaceus	5 liang
白芍	bái sháo	Root of Paeonia lactiflora	5 liang
白術	bái zhú	Rhizome of Atractylodes macrocephala	5 liang
山萸	shān yú	Fruit of Cornus officinalis	4 liang
人三	rén sān	Root of Panax ginseng	3 liang
茯苓	fú líng	Dried fungus of Poria cocos	3 liang
五味子	wǔ wèi zǐ	Fruit of Schisandra chinensis	3 liang
麥冬	mài dōng	Tuber of Ophiopogon japonicus	3 liang
神麴	shén qū	Medicated leaven	1 liang
砂仁	shā rén	Fruit of Amomum villosum	5 qian
陳皮	chén pí	Peel of Citrus reticulata	5 qian
當歸	dāng guī	Root of Angelica polimorpha	0.5 jin

Honeyed pills; take five qian each time with boiling water for twice a day, at dawn and at dusk.

日重夜輕

病重於日間，而發寒發熱，較夜尤重，此證必須從天未明而先截之。方用：

人三、枳殼、青皮、陳皮、半夏、甘草各壹錢，黃耆、白術各伍錢，當歸、柴胡各三錢，乾薑五分，水煎服。又方：

熟地壹兩，人三、陳皮、白芥子、甘草各壹錢，白術伍錢，柴胡貳錢，水煎服。

Seriousness in Daytime with Relief at Night

Symptoms are more badly felt during the day with severe fever or chill. It must be stopped before the dawn. Formula:

人三	rén sān	Root of Panax ginseng	1 qian
枳殼	zhǐ ké	Dried peel of Aurantii fructus	1 qian
青皮	qīng pí	Immature peel of Citrus reticulate	1 qian
陳皮	chén pí	Peel of Citrus reticulata	1 qian
半夏	bàn xià	Rhizome of Pinellia ternata	1 qian
甘草	gān cǎo	Root of Glycyrrhiza uralensis	1 qian
黃耆	huáng qí	Root of Astragalus membranaceus	5 qian
白術	bái zhú	Rhizome of Atractylodes macrocephala	5 qian
當歸	dāng guī	Root of Angelica polimorpha	3 qian

柴胡	chái hú	Root of Bupleurum chinense	3 qian
乾薑	gān jiāng	Dried root of Zingiber officinale	5 fen

Another formula:

熟地	shú dì	Prepared root of Rehmannia glutinosa	1 liang
人三	rén sān	Root of Panax ginseng	1 qian
陳皮	chén pí	Peel of Citrus reticulata	1 qian
白芥子	bái jièzĭ	Seed of Brassica alba	1 qian
甘草	gān căo	Root of Glycyrrhiza uralensis	1 qian
白術	bái zhú	Rhizome of Atractylodes macrocephala	5 qian
柴胡	chái hú	Root of Bupleurum chinense	2 qian

夜重日輕

病重於夜間，而發熱發寒，或寒少熱多，或熱少寒多，一到天明，便覺清爽，一到黃昏，即覺沉重，此陰氣虛甚也。方用：

熟地壹兩，山萸肆錢，當歸、白芍、柴胡、生何首烏、麥冬、白芥子各三錢、鱉甲，伍錢五味子，陳皮各壹錢，水煎服。

此方妙在用鱉甲乃至陰之物，逢陰則入，遇陽則轉；生何首烏直入陰經，亦攻邪氣；白芥子去痰，又不耗真陰之氣，有不奏功者乎？必須將黃昏時服，則陰氣固，而邪氣不敢入矣。

Seriousness at Night with Relief in Daytime

The disease predominates at night with symptoms of fever or chill, whether more times of fever and less chill or vice versa which are greatly relieved by dawn and become serious at dusk. This is due to the uttermost yin deficiency. Formula:

熟地 shú dì Prepared root of Rehmannia glutinosa 1 liang

山萸 shān yú Fruit of Cornus officinalis 4 qian

當歸 dāng guī Root of Angelica polimorpha 3 qian

白芍 bái sháo Root of Paeonia lactiflora 3 qian

柴胡 chái hú Root of Bupleurum chinense 3 qian

生何首烏 shēng hé shǒu wū Fresh root of Polygonum multiflorum 3 qian

麥冬 mài dōng Tuber of Ophiopogon japonicus 3 qian

白芥子 bái jiè zǐ Seed of Brassica alba 3 qian

鱉甲 biē jiǎ Dorsal shell of Amyda sinensis 5 qian

五味子 wǔ wèi zǐ Fruit of Schisandra chinensis 1 qian

陳皮 chén pí Peel of Citrus reticulata 1 qian

The formula's genius lies in its use of **biē jiǎ**, a yin medicinal which enters when coming across yin and *converse*[52] while encountering yang; **Shēng hé shǒu wū** enters into the yin meridians directly to attack pathogenic qi4; **Bái jiè zǐ** *dispels phlegm*[53] without consuming qi4 of the true yin. How could the formula fail? Patient must take the decoction by dusk in order that yin qi4 is secured and pathogenic qi4 dare not invade.

陰邪兼陽邪

此證亦發於夜間，亦發寒發熱，無異純陰邪氣之證，但少少煩燥耳，不若陰證之常靜也。法當於補陰之中，少加陽藥一二味，使陽長陰消，自奏功如響矣。方用：

熟地貳兩，山萸肆錢，鱉甲、茯苓各伍錢，當歸、白術、白芥子、麥冬、五味子、生何首烏各三錢，人三、柴胡各貳錢，陳皮壹錢，水煎服。

---

52 *converse*: yin-yang conversation, the property of the same entity can be transformed between yin and yang, also called inter-transformation of yin and yang.

53 *dispel phlegm*: a general term for therapeutic measures to treat phlegm pattern /syndrome, such as resolving phlegm or eliminating phlegm.

Concurrent Yin and Yang Pathogens

This syndrome also occurs in the evening with fever and chills. It is similar to syndromes of pure yin pathogenic qi4, except for a symptom of slight fidgeting of the patients, which is unlike the yin diseases characterized by the quietness of patients. Proper prescription is to add one or two yang-tonifying medicinals into the yin-tonifying ones, which helps with *yang waxing and yin waning*[54] and the cure is made. Formula:

熟地	shú dì	Prepared root of Rehmannia glutinosa	2 liang
山萸	shān yú	Fruit of Cornus officinalis	4 qian
鱉甲	biē jiǎ	Dorsal shell of Amyda sinensis□	5 qian
茯苓	fú líng	Dried fungus of Poria cocos	5 qian
當歸	dāng guī	Root of Angelica polimorpha	3 qian
白術	bái zhú	Rhizome of Atractylodes macrocephala	3 qian
白芥子	bái jiè zǐ	Seed of Brassica alba	3 qian
麥冬	mài dōng	Tuber of Ophiopogon japonicus	3 qian
五味子	wǔ wèi zǐ	Fruit of Schisandra chinensis	3 qian

---

[54] *yang waxing and yin waning*: alternation of strength and prevalence between the paired yin and yang, the same as natural flux of yin and yang or inter-consuming-supporting relationship of yin and yang.

生何首烏 shēng hé shǒu wū Fresh Root of Polygonum multiflorum 3 qian

人三 rén sān Root of Panax ginseng 2 qian

柴胡 chái hú Root of Bupleurum chinense 2 qian

陳皮 chén pí Peel of Citrus reticulate 1 qian

氣血兩虛

飲食不進，形容枯稿，補其氣，血益燥；補其血，氣益餒；助胃氣而盜汗難止，補血脈而胸膈阻滯，法當氣血同治。方用：

人三、白術、川芎、穀芽各壹錢，麥冬伍錢，甘草捌分，當歸、茯苓各貳錢，熟地、白芍各三錢，陳皮、神曲各伍分，水煎服。

此治氣血兩補，與八珍湯同功，而勝於八珍湯者，妙在補中有調和之法耳。

Dual Deficiency of Qi4 and Blood

Symptoms of *dual deficiency of qi4 and blood*[55] include inability of food and drink intake and a face as dry as

[55] *dual deficiency of qi4 and blood*: simultaneous presence of qi4 deficiency and blood deficiency.

parchment. If only qi4 is supplemented, blood will become drier; If only blood is supplemented, qi4 will be more frustrated; Night sweating is unquenchable if stomach qi4 is assisted, and the chest and diaphragm are felt obstructed if blood vessel is supplemented. Simultaneous treatment of both qi4 and blood is recommended. Formula:

人三	rén sān	Root of Panax ginseng	1 qian
白術	bái zhú	Rhizome of Atractylodes macrocephala	1 qian
川芎	chuān xiōng	Root of Ligusticum wallichii	1 qian
穀芽	gǔ yá	Sprout of Oryza sativa	1 qian
麥冬	mài dōng	Tuber of Ophiopogon japonicus	5 qian
甘草	gān cǎo	Root of Glycyrrhiza uralensis	8 fen
當歸	dāng guī	Root of Angelica polimorpha	2 qian
茯苓	fú líng	Dried fungus of Poria cocos	2 qian
熟地	shú dì	Prepared root of Rehmannia glutinosa	3 qian
白芍	bái sháo	Root of Paeonia lactiflora	3 qian
陳皮	chén pí	Peel of Citrus reticulata	5 fen
神麴	shén qū	Medicated leaven	5 fen

This treatment of tonifying both qi4 and blood is similar to *Ba Zhen Tang* in potency, but the advantage lies in its incorporation of both coordination and tonification.

氣虛胃虛

人有病久而氣虛者，必身體羸弱，飲食不進，或大便溏泄，小便艱澀。方用：

人三壹兩，白術伍錢，茯苓三錢，甘草、陳皮、車前子、澤瀉各壹錢，水煎服。

此方用人三為君者開其胃氣，蓋胃為腎之關，關門不開，則上之飲食不能進，下之糟粕不能化。必用人三以養胃土，茯苓車前以分消水氣。如服此不效，兼服八味丸，最能實大腸而利膀胱也。

Deficiency of Qi4 and Stomach

Patients of chronic disease normally have qi4 deficiency and weakness. They have difficulty in drinking and food intake, or they may have sloppy stools and rough urination. Formula:

人三	rén sān	Root of Panax ginseng	1 liang
白術	bái zhú	Rhizome of Atractylodes macrocephala	5 qian
茯苓	fú líng	Dried fungus of Poria cocos	3 qian
甘草	gān cǎo	Root of Glycyrrhiza uralensis	1 qian
陳皮	chén pí	Peel of Citrus reticulata	1 qian
車前子	chē qián zǐ	Seed of Plantago asiatica	1 qian
澤瀉	zé xiè	Rhizome of Alisma plantago-aquatica	1 qian

This formula employs **rén sān** as the monarch to open patient's stomach qi4. Since stomach is the pass to kidney, if the pass is closed, food and drink can not enter, nor can any dregs be transformed. **Rén sān** must be used to nourish the stomach earth, and **fú líng** and **chē qián zǐ** drain the water qi4. If this formula is not effective enough, patient can take *Ba Wei Wan* additionally to fortify the large intestines and faciliate the bladder.

氣虛飲食不消

飲食入胃，必須氣充足，始能消化而生津液，今飲食不消，氣虛也。方用：

人三貳錢，黃耆、白術、茯苓、甘草各三錢，神曲、麥芽、陳皮各伍分，山查三個，水煎服。

傷面食加來服子；有痰加半夏、白芥子各一錢；咳嗽加蘇子一錢，桔梗二錢；傷風加柴胡二錢；夜臥不安，加炒棗仁二錢；胸中微痛，加枳殼五分。方內純是開胃之品，又恐飲食難消，後加消導之品，則飲食化而津液生矣。

Indigestion Due to Qi4 Deficiency

People must have an adequate amount of qi4 inorder to transform and digest food, and to engender *fluid and humor*[56]. Indigestion is due to qi4 deficiency. Formula:

人三	rén sān	Root of Panax ginseng	2 qian
黄耆	huáng qí	Root of Astragalus membranaceus	3qian
白術	bái zhú	Rhizome of Atractylodes macrocephala	3 qian
茯苓	fú líng	Dried fungus of Poria cocos	3 qian
甘草	gān cǎo	Root of Glycyrrhiza uralensis	3 qian
神麴	shén qū	Medicated leaven	5 fen
麥芽	mài yá	Sprout of Oryza sativa	5 fen
陳皮	chén pí	Peel of Citrus reticulata	5 fen

[56] *fluid and humor:* a general term for all kinds of normal fluid in the body, except the blood, also known as body fluids.

山査　shān zhā　Fruit of Crateagus pinnatifida　3 pcs.

For *food damage*[57] due to food of flour, add **lái fú zǐ**; If there is phlegm, add one qian of **bàn xià** and one qian of **bái jiè zǐ**; For cough, add one qian of **sū zǐ** and two qian of **jié gěng**; For wind damage, add two qian of **chái hú**; For insomnia, add two qian of **chǎo zǎo rén;** For slight chest pain, add five fen of **zhǐ ké.** The medicinals of this formula just open the stomach of patient, but *digestant medicinals*[58] must be applied later to help with digestion in order to engender fluid and humor.

血虛面色黃瘦

出汗，盜汗，夜臥常醒，不能潤色以養筋是也。血虛自當補血，舍四物湯又何求耶？今不用四物湯。用：

熟地壹兩，麥冬、枸杞各三錢，當歸伍錢，茜草壹錢，桑葉拾片，水煎服。

---

[57] *food damage*: any disease of damage to the spleen and stomach by food.

[58] *digestant medicinals:* medicinals that aids digestion to eliminate accumulated undigested food.

此方妙在用桑葉以補陰而生血，又妙在加茜草，則血得活而益生，況又濟之歸、地、麥冬大劑，以共生乎！

Sallow-thin Complexion with Blood Deficiency

Symptoms of sweating, night sweating, and disturbed sleep are the results of failure in sinews' moistening and nourisment. For blood deficiency, blood-tonifying *Si Wu Tang* is generally prescribed. But here we recommend another formula:

熟地	shú dì	Prepared root of Rehmannia glutinosa	1 liang
麥冬	mài dōng	Tuber of Ophiopogon japonicus	3 qian
枸杞	gǒu qǐ	Fruit of Lycium chinensis	3 qian
當歸	dāng guī	Root of Angelica polimorpha	5 qian
茜草	qiàn cǎo□	Root of Rubia Cordifolia	1 qian
桑葉	sāng yè	Foliage of Mori	10 pcs.

The genius of this formula first of all lies in its use of **sāng yè** to supplement yin and engender blood. Secondly, **qiàn cǎo** activates and enlivens the blood. Moreover, the formula contains large doses of **dāng guī**, **shú dì,** and **mài dōng**, all of which are well coordinated.

肺脾雙虧

咳嗽不已，吐瀉不已，此肺脾受傷也。人以咳嗽宜治肺，吐瀉宜治脾。殊不知咳嗽由於脾氣之衰，斡旋之令不行，則上為咳嗽矣；吐瀉由於肺氣之弱，清肅之令不行，始上吐而下瀉矣。方用：

人三壹錢伍分，麥冬、茯苓各貳錢，車前子、甘草各壹錢，柴胡、神曲、薏仁各伍分，水煎服。

此治脾治肺之藥，合而用之咳嗽吐瀉之病各愈，所謂一方而兩用之也。

Dual Deficiency of Lung and Spleen

Incessant cough, helpless vomiting and diarrhea are symptoms of lung and spleen damage. While people know that lung is treated for coughing, and spleen is treated for vomiting and diarrhea, they do not know that cough is due to the debility of spleen qi4 and the failure of mediation, which goes up to be cough. Vomiting and diarrhea are due to weakness of lung qi4, which makes the clearing and clarification of pathogens infeasible, thus the suffering from vomiting and diarrhea. Formula:

人三	rén sān	Root of Panax ginseng	1 qian 5 fen
麥冬	mài dōng	Tuber of Ophiopogon japonicus	2 qian
茯苓	fú líng	Dried fungus of Poria cocos	2 qian
車前子	chē qián zǐ	Seed of Plantago asiatica	1 qian
甘草	gān cǎo	Root of Glycyrrhiza uralensis	1 qian
柴胡	chái hú	Root of Bupleurum chinense	5 fen
神麴	shén qū	Medicated leaven	5 fen
薏仁	yì rén	Seed kernel of Coix lachryma-jobi	5 fen

As a therapy for treating lung and spleen, the combined employment of the medicinals cures all of the coughing, vomiting and diarrhea, which is known as "to cure two diseases with one formula."

肝腎兩虛

腎水虧不能滋肝，則肝木抑鬱而不舒，必有兩脅飽悶之證；肝木不能生腎中之火，則腎水日寒，必有腰背難以服俯仰之證。此證必須肝腎同補。方用：

熟地壹兩，山萸、當歸、白芍各伍錢，柴胡貳錢，肉桂壹錢，水煎服。

熟地、山萸，補腎之藥，歸、芍、柴、桂，補肝之品，既雲平補，似乎用藥不宜有重輕，今補肝之藥多於補腎者何？蓋腎為肝之母，肝又為命門之母，豈有木旺而不生命門之火者哉？

Dual Deficiency of Liver and Kidney

When kidney water is depleted, liver cannot be enriched, which makes the liver wood despondent and tense, and the symptom of fullness and oppression on both sides of body is formed. If liver wood can not light kidney fire, the kidney water will be cooled down day by day, and patients will have difficulty in moving waists and backs. These symptoms must be treated by dual supplementation of both the liver and the kidney. Formula:

熟地	shú dì	Prepared root of Rehmannia glutinosa	1 liang
山萸	shān yú	Fruit of Cornus officinalis	5 qian
當歸	dāng guī	Root of Angelica polimorpha	5 qian
白芍	bái sháo	Root of Paeonia lactiflora	5 qian

柴胡	chái hú	Root of Bupleurum chinense	2 qian
肉桂	ròu guì	Bark of Cinnamonum cassia	1 qian

Shú dì and **shān yú** supplement the kidney; **Dāng guī**, **bái sháo**, **chái hú** and **ròu guì** supplement the liver. Normally with *neutral supplementation*[59], the dosages should be averaged. Why in this formula are there more herbs for supplementing liver than those for supplementing kidney? It is because kidney is the mother of liver, and liver is the mother of life gate. How can wood flourish when *life gate fire*[60] is not engendered?

心腎不交

腎，水藏也；心，火藏也；是心腎二經，為仇敵矣，似不可牽連而合治之也。不知心腎相克而實相須，腎無心之火則水寒，心無腎之水則火熾。心必得腎水以滋潤，腎必得心火以溫暖。如人驚惕不安，夢遺精泄，皆心腎不交之故。人以驚惕為心之病，我以為腎之病；人以夢泄為腎

[59] *neutral supplementation*: equal reinforcement by lifting and thrusting evenly with the same amplitude or rotation at a favorable angle, the same as neutral reinforcement.

[60] *life gate fire*: innate fire from the life gate, a synonym of kidney yang.

之病，我以為心之病；非顛倒也，實有至理焉。人果細心思之，自然明白。方用：

熟地、白術各伍兩，山萸、人三、茯神、棗仁炒、麥冬、柏子仁各三兩，遠志、菖蒲、五味子各壹兩，山藥三錢，芡實伍錢，蜜丸，每早、晚滬水送下五錢。

此方之妙，治腎之藥，少於治心之味，蓋心君謐靜，腎氣自安，何至心動？此治腎正所以治心，治心即所以治腎也，所謂心腎相依。

Failure in Communication between Heart and Kidney

Kidney accumulates water and heart accumulates fire. Thus, their meridians are often seen as enemies and it is impossible to treat them simultaneously. However, the relationship between heart and kidney is one of restraint in appearance and of *mutual reinforcement*[61] in nature. Kidney water if deprived of heart fire will be cooled down, and heart fire if without kidney water will blaze. Thus, heart must be enriched and moistened with kidney water, and kidney must be warmed by heart fire. The symptoms of constant vigilance

61 *mutual reinforcement*: two medicinals with similar properties used in combination to reinforce each other's action, or organs' reinforcement of each other.

and *dream emission*[62] are due to failure in communication between the heart and the kidney. People believe that sudden fright is a heart disease, but I think it is a kidney one; People think that dream emission is a kidney disease, but I believe it is a heart one. It is not my intentional inversion, but a firmly rooted fact. Readers will understand this prescription if to think twice. Formula

熟地 shú dì Prepared root of Rehmannia glutinosa 5 liang
白術 bái zhú Rhizome of Atractylodes macrocephala 5 liang
山萸 shān yú Fruit of Cornus officinalis 3 liang
人三 rén sān Root of Panax ginseng 3 liang
茯神 fú shén Sclerotium of Poria cocos 3 liang
棗仁炒zǎo rén chǎo Stir-fried seed of Ziziphus jujuba 3 liang
麥冬 mài dōng Tuber of Ophiopogon japonicus 3 liang
柏子仁 bǎi zǐ rén Seed of Platycladus orientalis 3 liang
遠志 yuǎn zhì Root of Polygala tenuifolia 1 liang
菖蒲 chāng pú Rhizome of Acorus gramineus 1 liang

---

62 *dream emission*: involuntary emission of semen during sleep associated with dreaming.

五味子 wǔ wèi zǐ Fruit of Schisandra chinensis 1 liang
山藥 shān yào Root of Dioscorea opposita 3 qian
芡實 qiàn shí Seed of Gordon Euryale 5 qian

Take five qian of honeyed pills twice a day in morning and evening with warm water.

The genius of this formula is that the medicinals treating kidney are less in doses than those treating the heart. If monarchic heart is quieted down, kidney qi4 will be settled. How can the heart fidget? Treating heart equals to treating kidney, and the vice versa is true. This is known as "interdependence between the heart and the kidney".

精滑夢遺

此證人以為腎虛也。不獨腎病也，心病也。宜心腎兼治。方用：

熟地半斤，山藥、肉桂、鹿茸、炒棗仁、遠志、杜仲、柏子仁、破故紙、五味子各壹兩，山萸、白術各肆兩，人三、茯苓、麥冬、白芍、巴戟、肉蓯蓉各三兩，紫河車壹副，砂仁伍錢，附子壹錢，蜜丸。早晚白水送下五錢。

此方用熟地、山藥、山萸之類，補腎也；巴戟、肉蓯蓉、附子、鹿茸，補腎中之火也，可以已矣。而又必加人三、茯苓、柏子仁、麥冬、遠志、棗仁者何也？蓋腎火虛由於心火虛也，使補腎火不補心火，則反增上焦枯渴，故欲補腎火，必須補心火，則水火相濟也。

Spermatorrhea[63] and Dream Emission

The syndrome is believed to be caused by kidney deficiency, though it is not merely a kidney disease but a heart one. It is appropriate to treat heart and kidney duly. Formula:

熟地 shú dì Prepared root of Rehmannia glutinosa 5 liang
山藥 shān yào Root of Dioscorea opposita 1 liang
肉桂 ròu guì Bark of Cinnamonum cassia 1 liang
鹿茸 lù róng Pilose antler of Cervus nippon 1 liang
炒棗仁 chǎo zǎo rén Stir-fried seed of Ziziphus jujuba1 liang
遠志 yuǎn zhì Root of Polygala tenuifolia 1 liang
杜仲 dù zhòng Bark of Eucommia ulmoidis 1 liang
柏子仁 bǎi zǐ rén Seed of Platycladus orientalis 1 liang

[63] *spermatorrhea*: involuntary and frequent discharge of semen without copulation.

破故紙 pò gù zhǐ Foliage of Clammy Hopseedbush 1 liang
五味子 wǔ wèi zǐ Fruit of Schisandra chinensis 1 liang
山萸 shān yú Fruit of Cornus officinalis 4 liang
白術 bái zhú Rhizome of Atractylodes macrocephala 4 liang
人三 rén sān Root of Panax ginseng 3 liang
茯苓 fú líng Dried fungus of Poria cocos 3 liang
麥冬 mài dōng Tuber of Ophiopogon japonicus 3 liang
白芍 bái sháo Root of Paeonia lactiflora 3 liang
巴戟 bā jǐ Root of Morinda officinalis 3 liang
肉蓯蓉 ròu cōng róng Fleshy stalk of Cistanche salsa 3 liang
紫河車 zǐ hé chē Dried Human Placenta 1 piece
砂仁 shā rén Fruit of Amomum villosum 5 qian
附子 fù zǐ Lateral root of Aconitum carmichaeli 1 qian

Take five qian of honeyed pills twice a day, in morning and in evening with boiled water.

The formula uses **shú dì**, **shān yào,** and **shān yú** to supplement the kidney, and **bā jǐ**, **ròu cōng róng**, **fù zǐ**, **lù róng** to supplement kidney fire. That is quite enough. Why must **rén sān, fú líng, bǎi zǐ rén, mài dōng, yuǎn zhì**, and **zǎo rén** be added? It is because that deficiency of kidney fire is due to deficiency of heart fire, and the supplementation of kidney fire, if without supplementing heart fire, will make the upper energizer parched and thirsty. Therefore, to supplement kidney fire, heart fire must be supplemented as well. Only in this way can the fire and the water benefit each other.

夜夢遺精

此證由於腎水耗竭，上不能通於心，中不能潤於肝，下不生於脾，以致玉關不閉，無夢且遺。法當補腎而少佐以益心、肝、脾之品。方用：

熟地壹兩，山萸肆錢，茯苓、白芍、生棗仁、當歸、薏仁各三錢，白術伍錢，茯神貳錢，五味子、白芥子各壹錢，肉桂、黃連各伍分，水煎服。

一劑止，十劑不犯。

Night Dreams and Incontinence of Seminal Fluid

Exhausted kidney water can neither ascend to the heart of upper body, moisten the liver of middle, nor can it descend to connect to the spleen of lower body. As a result, the jade pass is left open and the incontinence of seminal fluid is made even when without dreams. It is a proper therapy to tonify kidney with assistance of medicinals benefitting heart, liver, and spleen. Formula:

熟地 shú dì Prepared root of Rehmannia glutinosa 1 liang
山萸 shān yú Fruit of Cornus officinalis 4 qian
茯苓 fú líng Dried fungus of Poria cocos 3 qian
白芍 bái sháo Root of Paeonia lactiflora 3 qian
生棗仁 shēng zǎo rén Fresh seed of Ziziphus jujuba 3 qian
當歸 dāng guī Root of Angelica polimorpha 3 qian
薏仁 yì rén Seed kernel of Coix lachryma-jobi 3 qian
白術 bái zhú Rhizome of Atractylodes macrocephala 5 qian
茯神 fú shén Sclerotium of Poria cocos 2 qian
五味子 wǔ wèi zǐ Fruit of Schisandra chinensis 1 qian
白芥子 bái jiè zǐ Seed of Brassica alba 1 qian
肉桂 ròu guì Bark of Cinnamonum cassia 5 fen
黃連 huáng lián Rhizome of Coptis chinensis 5 fen

One dose stops the syndrome and in ten doses it is cured.

遺精健忘

遺精，下病；健忘，上病也；何以合治之而鹹當乎？蓋遺精雖是腎水之虛，而實本於君火之弱，今補其心君，則玉關不必閉而自閉矣，所謂一舉而兩得也。方用：

人三、茯實、麥冬、生棗仁、當歸、山萸各三兩，蓮須貳兩，熟地伍兩，山藥肆兩，柏子仁去油、遠志、昌蒲、五味子各壹兩，蜜丸。每日服五錢，白水下。

Incontinence of Seminal Fluid and Forgetfulness

Incontinence of Seminal Fluid is a disease of the lower body, while *forgetfulness*[64] is one of the upper. How can they be properly treated simultaneously? Dream emission is in nature rooted in the heart fire deficiency though apparently a kidney water deficiency symptom. If heart is supplemented, the jade pass will close by itself. This is to kill two birds with one stone. Formula:

---

[64] *forgetfulness*: poor memory; tendency to forget matters, the same as amnesia.

人三 rén sān Root of Panax ginseng 3 liang

芡實 qiàn shí□ Seed of Gordon Euryale 3 liang

麥冬 mài dōng Tuber of Ophiopogon japonicas 3 liang

生棗仁 shēng zǎo rén Fresh seed of Ziziphus jujube 3 liang

當歸 dāng guī Root of Angelica polimorpha 3 liang

山萸 shān yú Fruit of Cornus officinalis 3 liang

蓮須 lián xū Lotus Stamen 2 liang

熟地 shú dì Prepared root of Rehmannia glutinosa 5 liang

山藥 shān yào Root of Dioscorea opposita 4 liang

柏子仁(去油) bǎi zǐ rén Seed of Platycladus orientalis (deoiled) 1 liang

遠志 yuǎn zhì Root of Polygala tenuifolia 1 liang

菖蒲 chāng pú Rhizome of Acorus gramineus 1 liang

五味子 wǔ wèi zǐ Fruit of Schisandra chinensis 1 liang

Take five qian of honeyed pills daily with boiled water.

倒飽中滿

氣虛不能食，食則倒滿。方用：

人三、來服子、甘草各壹錢，白術貳錢，茯苓、山藥各三錢，芡實、薏仁各五錢，陳皮三分，水煎服。

下喉雖則微脹，入腹漸覺爽快。

Stomach Distention and Fullness in the Middle

Patients with qi4 deficiency can not have food. Food intake gives them a feeling of complete fullness. Formula:

人三	rén sān	Root of Panax ginseng	1 qian
來服子	lái fú zĭ	Radish Seed	1 qian
甘草	gān căo	Root of Glycyrrhiza uralensis	1 qian
白術	bái zhú	Rhizome of Atractylodes macrocephala	2 qian
茯苓	fú líng	Dried fungus of Poria cocos	3 qian
山藥	shān yào	Root of Dioscorea opposita	3 qian
芡實	qiàn shí□	Seed of Gordon Euryale	5 qian
薏仁	yì rén	Seed kernel of Coix lachryma-jobi	5 qian
陳皮	chén pí	Peel of Citrus reticulata	3 fen

Fullness is felt upon drinking the decoction, but ease is felt gradually afterwards.

久虛緩補

久虛之人，氣息奄奄，無不曰宜急治矣。不知氣血大虛，驟加大補之劑，力量難任，必致胃口轉膨脹，不如緩緩清補之也。方用：

當歸、茯苓、山藥各壹錢，白芍貳錢，白術、棗仁各伍分，人三、陳皮、麥芽、炮薑、甘草各三分，水煎服。

此方妙在以白芍為君，引三、苓入肝為佐，小小使令徐徐奏功。使脾氣漸實，胃口漸開，然後再用純補之劑，先宜緩補之也。如久餓之人驟投以飯則飽死，須以薄粥徐徐飲之，同是一理。

Gradual Tonification for Chronic Deficiency

All professionals prescribe emergent treatment to those who are dying of chronic deficiency. However, they have no idea that patients with serious qi4 and blood deficiency if tonified with strong doses, can not endure the mecicinal strength and their stomachs will distend. A better solution is to use gradual moistening tonification. Formula:

當歸	dāng guī	Root of Angelica polimorpha	1 qian
茯苓	fú líng	Dried fungus of Poria cocos	1 qian

山藥	shān yà	Root of Dioscorea opposita	1 qian
白芍	bái sháo	Root of Paeonia lactiflora	2 qian
白術	bái zhú	Rhizome of Atractylodes macrocephala	5 fen
棗仁	zǎo rén	Seed of Ziziphus jujuba	5 fen
人三	rén sān	Root of Panax ginseng	3 fen
陳皮	chén pí	Peel of Citrus reticulata	3 fen
麥芽	mài yá	Sprout of Oryza sativa	3 fen
炮薑	pào jiāng	Sand-fried Common ginger	3 fen
甘草	gān cǎo	Root of Glycyrrhiza uralensis	3 fen

The genius of this formula lies in its use of **bái sháo** as monarch with **rén sān** and **fú líng** as assistants in guiding strength into the liver. Moderate medicament leads to a gradual cure by fortifying spleen qi4 and increasing patients' appetite, and then it uses refined tonifying medicinals to tonify gradually. An extremely hungry person when sated with abundant food may die of fullness. Instead, he should be given thin porridge slowly. The same is true here.

補氣

右手脈大，氣分之勞也。方用補氣丸：

人三、黃耆、白芍各三兩，茯苓肆兩，白術半斤，陳皮、五味子、白芥子、遠志各壹兩，麥冬貳兩，炙甘草捌分，蜜丸。早服五錢，白水下。

Qi4 Tonification

Strong right hand pulse is a symptom of *qi4 aspect*[65] consumption. The formula is *Bu Qi Wan* [pinyin: bǔ qì wán, 補氣丸, Qi4 Tonification Pill]:

人三	rén sān	Root of Panax ginseng	3 liang
黃耆	huáng qí	Root of Astragalus membranaceus	3 liang
白芍	bái sháo	Root of Paeonia lactiflora	3 liang
茯苓	fú líng	Dried fungus of Poria cocos	4 liang
白術	bái zhú	Rhizome of Atractylodes macrocephala	5 liang
陳皮	chén pí	Peel of Citrus reticulata	1 liang
五味子	wǔ wèi zǐ	Fruit of Schisandra chinensis	1 liang
白芥子	bái jiè zi	Seed of Brassica alba (L.) Boiss.	1 liang
遠志	yuǎn zhì	Root of Polygala tenuifolia	1 liang

[65] qi4 *aspect*: the second stratum of the body deeper than the defense aspect, often referring to the lung, gallbladder, spleen, stomach, and large intestine.

麥冬 mài dōng Tuber of Ophiopogon japonicas 2 liang
炙甘草 jiù gān cǎo Prepared root of Glycyrrhiza uralensis 8 fen

Take five qian of honeyed pills in morning with boiled water.

補血

左手脈大，血分之勞也。方用補血丸：

熟地、白芍各半斤，山萸、當歸各肆兩，棗仁、麥冬、白芥子、五味子壹兩，砂仁、肉桂各伍錢，蜜丸。

晚服一兩，白水下，如身熱，去肉桂，加地骨皮五錢。

Blood Tonification

A strong left hand pulse indicates blood aspect consumption. The formula is *Bu Xue Wan* [pinyin: bǔ xuè wán, 補血丸, Blood Tonification Pill]:

熟地 shú dì Prepared root of Rehmannia glutinosa half jin
白芍 bái sháo Root of Paeonia lactiflora half hu
山萸 shān yú Fruit of Cornus officinalis 4 liang
當歸 dāng guī Root of Angelica polimorpha 4 liang

棗仁	zǎo rén	Seed of Ziziphus jujuba	1 qian
麥冬	mài dōng	Tuber of Ophiopogon japonicus	1 qian
白芥子	bái jiè zǐ	Seed of Brassica alba	1 qian
五味子	wǔ wèi zǐ	Fruit of Schisandra chinensis	1 liang
砂仁	shā rén	Fruit of Amomum villosum	5 qian
肉桂	ròu guì	Bark of Cinnamonum cassia	5 qian

Take one liang of honeyed pills in evening with boiled water. If there is fever, remove **ròu guì** from the formula, and add five qian of **dì gǔ pí**.

出汗

人有病不宜汗多，若過出汗，恐其亡陽，不可不用藥以斂之。方用：

人三、黃芪、當歸各壹兩，桑葉伍片，麥冬三錢，炒棗仁壹錢，水煎服。

Sweating

Patients should not sweat excessively. Too much of sweating may lead to *yang collapse*[66]. The prescription is to stop sweating. Formula:

人三	rén sān	Root of Panax ginseng	1 liang
黃耆	huáng qí	Root of Astragalus membranaceus	1 liang
當歸	dāng guī	Root of Angelica polimorpha	1 liang
桑葉	sāng yè	Foliage of Mori	5 pcs.
麥冬	mài dōng	Tuber of Ophiopogon japonicus	3 qian
炒棗仁	chǎo zǎo rén	Stir-fried seed of Ziziphus jujuba	1 qian

痨證

痨證既成，最難治者，必有蟲生之，以食人之氣血也。若徒補其氣血，而不入殺蟲之藥，則飲食入胃，衹蔭蟲而不生氣血。若但殺蟲而不補氣血，則五藏俱受傷，又何有生理哉？惟於大補之中，加殺蟲之藥，則元氣既全，真陽未散，蟲死而身安矣。方用 ：

熟地、地栗粉、何首烏各半斤，鱉甲、山藥各壹斤，

66 *yang collapse*: a pathological change where yang qi4 is suddenly exhausted, resulting in abrupt failure of bodily functions.

神麴、麥冬各伍兩，桑葉半斤，人參、白微各參兩，熟地為丸。

每日白水送下五錢，半年蟲從大便出矣。

Consumptive Symptoms

Consumption, once befallen, is the hardest to tackle. Worms must have grown to eat patients' qi4 and blood. If only qi4 and blood tonification is applied without killing the worms, digested food in stomach will only nourish the worms instead of engendering qi4 and blood. But if the worms are killed without tonifying qi4 and blood, the five viscera will be damaged, and how can patients be saved? Simultaneous tonification and worm killing will bring about the culmination of complete source qi4, intact genuine yang, and the death of worms. Formula:

熟地	shú dì	Prepared root of Rehmannia glutinosa	half jin
地栗粉	dì lì fěn	Powder of Waternut corm	half jin
何首烏	hé shŏu wū	Tuber of multiflower knotweed	half jin
鱉甲	biē jiă	Dorsal shell of Amyda sinensis	1 jin
山藥	shān yào	Root of Dioscorea opposita	1 jin

神麴	shén qū	Medicated leaven	5 liang
麥冬	mài dōng	Tuber of Ophiopogon japonicus	5 liang
桑葉	sāng yè	Foliage of Mori	half jin
人三	rén sān	Root of Panax ginseng	3 liang
白薇	bái wēi	Root of Cynanchum atratum	3 liang

Pills of the medicinals mixed with **shú dì** are to be taken five qian per day with boiled water. The worms will be out with feces in a time of six months.

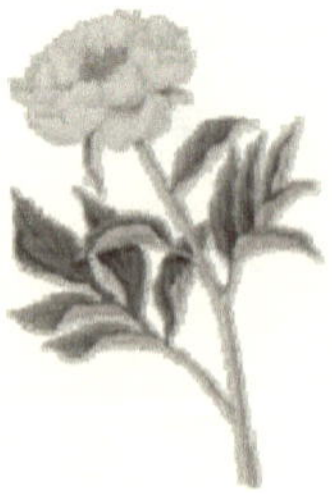

痰嗽門

Chapter 5 Phlegm & Cough

痰嗽

古人所立治痰之法，皆是治痰之標，而不能治其本也。如二陳湯，上、中、下、久、暫之痰皆治之，而其實無實效也。今立三方，痰病總不出其範圍也。

Phlegm & Cough

Ancient formulae for phlegm treatment all aim at treating the tip of phlegm instead of treating the root. For example, *Er Chen Tang* [pinyin: èr chén tāng, 二陳湯, Two Old Medicinals Decoction] treats chronic and temporary phlegm of whether the upper, middle or lower body, though in reality with no much effect. Three formulae are hereinafter given that cover all phlegm diseases.

初病之痰

傷風咳嗽，吐痰是也。方用：

陳皮、半夏、花粉、茯苓、蘇子、甘草各壹錢，水煎服。

二劑而痰可消矣。此去上焦之痰。上焦之痰，原在胃中而不在肺，去其胃中之痰，而肺金自然清肅，又何致火之上升哉？

此證醫治不善，極易成勞。緣痰嗽皆責之於肺，傷風痰嗽是風傷肺也。若發散燥痰太過，則肺不斂，必嗽愈甚，而上嗆血絲，久則肺傷而腎熾。若寒涼滋潤太過，則肺不舒必痰愈多，而氣喘聲痿，久則金冷而水寒。此方無此二弊，願病者勿以小病而忽之也。

Phlegm of Onset Diseases

Formula for wind-damage cough with expectoration:

陳皮	chén pí	Peel of Citrus reticulata	1 qian
半夏	bàn xià	Rhizome of Pinellia ternata	1 qian
花粉	huā fěn	Seed of Trichosanthes kirilowii	1 qian
茯苓	fú líng	Dried fungus of Poria cocos	1 qian
蘇子	sū zi zǐ	Seed of Perilla frutescens	1 qian
甘草	gān cǎo	Root of Glycyrrhiza uralensis	1 qian

Phlegm vanishes in two doses. This formula aims at removing phlegm of the upper energizer. Phlegm in upper energizer originates in stomach instead of the lung, if stomach phlegm is dispelled, the lung will be clear and cleansed naturally. How can the fire upraise?

If not properly treated, the syndrome may easily turn into a consumptive disease in that the lung is always blamed for phlegm and cough, and wind-damage cough with phlegm is caused by wind damage to the lung. If dry phlegm is over-dispersed, the lung can not be constrained and cough will develop, which causes slight blood sputum that damages the lung and blazes the kidney over time. If an excessive amount of cold, cool or moistenting medicinals are used, the constrained lung will have symptoms of more phlegm, panting and a lowered voice of patient, chronic case of which will lead to cold lung and chilled kidney. This formula, on the other hand, has no such defects. I hope that phlegm would not be underestimated as just a minor ailment.

已病之痰

必觀其色之白與黃而辨之，黃者火已退也，白者火正熾也。正熾者用寒涼之品，將退者用祛逐之味，今一方而俱治之。方用：

白朮、白芥子各叁錢，茯苓伍錢，陳皮、甘草各壹錢，枳殼伍分，水煎服。有火加梔子，無火不必加。此方健脾去溼，治痰之在中焦者也。又方：

白朮、茯苓、薏仁各五錢，人三五分，陳皮壹錢，天花粉貳錢，益智參分，水煎服。

有火加黃苓一錢；無火加乾薑一錢，甘草二分。此方健脾去溼而不耗氣，二劑而痰自消也。

Phlegm of Arisen Diseases

The color of phlegm must be observed in order to distinguish. Yellow phlegm indicates a retreated fire, while white phlegm means a blazing one. Blazing fire should be treated with cold and cool medicinals and retreating fire is dealt with medicinals of elimination and purgation. A formula tackling both is recommended here:

白朮	bái zhú	Rhizome of Atractylodes macrocephala	3 qian
白芥子	bái jiè zǐ	Seed of Brassica alba	3 qian
茯苓	fú líng	Dried fungus of Poria cocos	5 qian

陳皮	chén pí	Peel of Citrus reticulata	1 qian
甘草	gān cǎo	Root of Glycyrrhiza uralensis	1 qian
枳殼	zhǐ ké	Dried peel of Aurantii fructus	5 fen

If there is fire, add **zhī zǐ** into the formula and not to add if without. The formula fortifies spleen and eliminates dampness, treating phlegm of the middle energizer. Another formula:

白朮	bái zhú	Rhizome of Atractylodes macrocephala	5 qian
茯苓	fú líng	Dried fungus of Poria cocos	5 qian
薏仁	yì rén	Seed kernel of Coix lachryma-jobi	5 qian
人三	rén sān	Root of Panax ginseng	3 liang
陳皮	chén pí	Peel of Citrus reticulata	1 qian
天花粉	tiān huā fěn	Seed of Trichosanthes kirilowii	2 qian
益智	yì zhì	Fruit of Sharpleaf Galangal	3 fen

In case with fire, add one qian of **huáng qín**; in case without fire, add one qian of **gān jiāng** and two fen of **gān cǎo**. This formula fortifies spleen and eliminates the dampness while without consuming qi4. In two doses the phlegm will vanish.

久病之痰

久病痰多，切不可作脾溼生痰論之。蓋久病不愈，未有不因腎水虧損者也。非腎水泛上之痰，即腎火沸騰為痰，當補腎以袪逐之。方用：

熟地、薏仁各壹兩，山藥、山萸、麥冬、芡實各伍錢，五味子、茯苓各叁錢，益智仁貳錢，車前子壹錢，水煎服。

此治水泛為痰之聖藥也。若火沸騰為痰，加肉桂一錢，補腎去溼而化痰。水入腎宮，自變為真精而不化痰矣。此治下焦之痰也。又方：六味地黃湯，加麥冬、五味子，實有奇功。無火加桂、附。

Phlegm of Chronic Diseases

Excessive phlegm due to chronic disease should not be regarded as phlegm caused by spleen dampness. Patients with chronic diseases are normally suffers from kidney water deficiency. Phlegm is either made by upward flooding of kidney water or through boiling of kidney water by kidney fire. It is a proper treatment to tonify kidney and dispel phleghm. Formula:

熟地	shú dì	Prepared root of Rehmannia glutinosa	1 liang
薏仁	yì rén	Seed kernel of Coix lachryma-jobi	1 liang
山藥	shān yào	Root of Dioscorea opposita	5 qian
山萸	shān yú	Fruit of Cornus officinalis	5 qian
麥冬	mài dōng	Tuber of Ophiopogon japonicus	5 qian
芡實	qiàn shí□	Seed of Gordon Euryale	5 qian
五味子	wǔ wèi zǐ	Fruit of Schisandra chinensis	3 qian
茯苓	fú líng	Dried fungus of Poria cocos	3 qian
益智仁	yì zhì rén	Fruit of Sharpleaf Galangal	2 qian
車前子	chē qián zǐ	Seed of Plantago asiatica	1 qian

This is a magic remedy for water-flood phlegm. For phlegm due to the boiling of kidney water, add one qian of **ròu guì** to tonify the kidney, eliminate dampness and transform phlegm. Water returns into kidney to be *zhen jing* (真精, true essence) instead of phlegm. This treats phlegm of lower energizer. Another effective formula is *Liu Wei Di*

Huang Tang added with **mài dōng** and **wǔ wèi zǐ**. If without fire, add **fù zǐ** and **ròu guì**.

滯痰

夫痰之滯，乃氣之滯也。苟不補氣，而惟去其痰，未見痰去而病消也。方用：

人參、陳皮、花粉、白芥子各壹錢，白朮貳錢，茯苓叁錢，蘇子捌分，白蔻仁貳粒，水煎服。

Stagnated Phlegm

Stagnation of phlegm is in fact stagnation of qi4. If to eliminate phlegm without tonifying qi4, the phlegm will not vanish and the disease will not disappear. Formula:

人參	rén shēn	Root of Panax ginseng	1 qian
陳皮	chén pí	Peel of Citrus reticulata	1 qian
花粉	huā fěn	Seed of Trichosanthes kirilowii	1 qian
白芥子	bái jiè zǐ	Seed of Brassica alba	1 qian
白朮	bái zhú	Rhizome of Atractylodes macrocephala	2 qian
茯苓	fú líng	Dried fungus of Poria cocos	3 qian
蘇子	sū zǐ	Seed of Perilla frutescens	8 fen

白蔻仁	bái kòu rén	Cardamom	2 pcs.

溼痰

治痰之法，不可徒去其溼，必以補氣為先，而佐以化痰之品，乃克有效。方用：

人參壹兩，茯苓、半夏、神麴各叁錢，薏仁伍錢，陳皮、甘草各壹錢，水煎服。

蓋此方之中用神麴，人多不識，謂神麴乃消食之味，絕非化痰之品。不知痰之積聚稠粘，甚不易化，惟用此神麴以發之，則積聚稠粘開矣，繼之以半夏、陳皮，可以奏功。然雖有陳、半消痰，使不多用人參，則痰難消。今有人參以助氣，又有薏仁、茯苓，健脾去溼，而痰焉有不消者乎？

Damp Phlegm

Effectiveness of phlegm treatment consists not in the elimination of dampness, but in the tonification of qi4 assisted by medicinals transforming phlegm. Formula:

人參	rén shēn	Root of Panax ginseng	1 liang
茯苓	fú líng	Dried fungus of Poria cocos	3 qian

半夏	bàn xià	Rhizome of Pinellia ternata	3 qian
神麴	shén qū	Medicated leaven	3 qian
薏仁	yì rén	Seed kernel of Coix lachryma-jobi	5 qian
陳皮	chén pí	Peel of Citrus reticulata	1 qian
甘草	gān cǎo	Root of Glycyrrhiza uralensis	1 qian

The employment of **shén qū** in this formula is rarely understood by people, who claim that **shén qū** is for indigestion, not for phlegm transformation. They do not know that the accumulated phlegm, thick and sticky, is extremely difficult to transform. Only by using **shén qū** to develop the phlegm, can the accumulated phlegm be thinned and openned. And the addition of **bàn xià** and **chén pí** lands in success. Even when **bàn xià** and **chén pí** are added, the phlegm is difficult to clear if without the assistance of **rén shēn**. **Rén shēn** assists qi4, **yì rén** and **fú líng** fortity the spleen and eliminate dampness. How can the phlegm stay?

寒痰

人有氣虛而痰寒者，即用前方加肉桂三錢、乾薑五分足之矣。

Cold Phlegm

It is enough to use the above formula with an additional three qian of **ròu guì** and five fen of **gān jiāng** for patients with *cold phlegm syndrome*[67] due to qi4 deficiency,

熱痰

人有氣虛而痰熱者。方用：

當歸叁錢，白芍、麥冬、茯苓各貳錢，甘草、白芥子、花粉、陳皮各壹錢，神麴參分，水煎服。

Heat Phlegm

Formula for patients with *heat-phlegm syndrome*[68] due to qi4 deficiency

---

[67] *cold-phlegm pattern/syndrome*: a pattern/syndrome marked by cough with whitish expectoration, dyspnea or wheezing, aversion to cold with cold limbs, white slimy tongue coating, and wiry slippery or tense pulse.

[68] *heat-phlegm pattern/syndrome*: a pattern/syndrome arising when turbid phlegm combined with pathogenic heat accumulates in the lung and harasses the heart, marked by cough with yellowish expectoration, vexing stuffiness in the chest, fever, thirst, palpitations, insomnia, short voidings of deep-colored urine, reddened tongue with yellow greasy slimy coating and rapid slippery pulse.

當歸	dāng guī	Root of Angelica polimorpha	3 qian
白芍	bái sháo	Root of Paeonia lactiflora	2 qian
麥冬	mài dōng	Tuber of Ophiopogon japonicus	2 qian
茯苓	fú líng	Dried fungus of Poria cocos	2 qian
甘草	gān cǎo	Root of Glycyrrhiza uralensis	1 qian
白芥子	bái jiè zǐ	Seed of Brassica alba	1 qian
花粉	huā fěn	Seed of Trichosanthes kirilowii	1 qian
陳皮	chén pí	Peel of Citrus reticulata	1 qian
神麴	shén qū	Medicated leaven	3 fen

老痰

凡痰在胸膈不化者，謂之老痰。方用：

柴胡、茯苓、甘草、陳皮、丹皮、花粉各壹錢，白芍、薏仁各壹錢，白芥子伍錢，水煎服。

此方妙在百芥子為君，薏仁、白芍為臣，柴胡、花粉為佐，使老痰無處可藏，十劑而老痰可化矣。

Lingering Phlegm

Phlegm, in chest and diaphragm which cannot be transformed, is called lingering phlegm. Formula:

柴胡	chái hú	Root of Bupleurum chinense	1 qian

茯苓 fú líng Dried fungus of Poria cocos 1 qian

甘草 gān cǎo Root of Glycyrrhiza uralensis 1 qian

陳皮 chén pí Peel of Citrus reticulata 1 qian

丹皮 dān pí Bark of the root of Paeonia suffruticosa 1 qian

花粉 huā fěn Seed of Trichosanthes kirilowii 1 qian

白芍 bái sháo Root of Paeonia lactiflora 1 qian

薏仁 yì rén Seed kernel of Coix lachryma-jobi 1 qian□

百芥子 bái jiè zǐSeed of Brassica alba 5 qian

The genius of this formula lies in its use of **bǎi jiè zǐ** as sovereign with **yì rén** and **bái sháo** as ministers and **chái hú** and **huā fěn** as assistants. This combination renders the lingering phlegm nowhere to hide, and it will be transformed in ten doses.

頑痰

痰成而塞咽喉者，謂之頑痰。方用 ：

貝母、半夏、茯苓各叄錢，白朮伍錢，神麯貳錢，甘草、桔梗、白礬、炙紫苑各壹錢，水煎服。

此方妙在貝母、半夏同用，一燥一溼，使痰無處逃避；又有白礬消塊，梗、苑去邪，甘草調中，有不奏功者乎？

Stubborn Phlegm

Phlegm that forms in and obstructs the throat is called stubborn phlegm. Formula:

貝母	bèi mǔ	Bulb of Fritillaria cirrhosa	3 qian
半夏	bàn xià	Rhizome of Pinellia ternata	3 qian
茯苓	fú líng	Dried fungus of Poria cocos	3 qian
白朮	bái zhú	Rhizome of Atractylodes macrocephala	5 qian
神麴	shén qū	Medicated leaven	2 qian
甘草	gān cǎo	Root of Glycyrrhiza uralensis	1 qian
桔梗	jié gěng	Root of Platycodon grandiflorum	1 qian
白礬	bái fán	Alumen	1 qian
炙紫菀	zhì zǐ yuàn	Prepared root and rhizome of Aster tataricus	1 qian

The formula's genius lies in its combined use of **bèi mǔ** and **bàn xià**, one is dry in property and the other is wet, which leaves the phlegm nowhere to hide. Moreover, **bái fán** dissolves lumps, **jié gěng** and **zhì zǐ yuàn** dispel pathogens while **gān cǎo** harmonizes the middle. How could the formula not succeed?

水泛為痰

腎中之水，有火則安，無火則泛。倘人過於入房，則水去而火亦去，久之則水虛而火亦虛，水無可藏之地，必泛上為痰矣。治之法，欲抑水之下降，必先使火之下溫。當於補腎之中，加大熱之藥，使水足以制火，火足以煖水，則水火有既濟之道，自不上泛為痰矣。方用 ：

熟地壹兩，山萸伍錢，肉桂貳錢，牛膝叁錢，五味子壹錢，水煎服。

一劑而痰下行矣，二劑而痰自消矣。

Phlegm Due to Water-flood

Kidney water is peaceful when there is fire, and will flood when without fire. If a man excessively indulges in sexual activity, his water and fire will both exhaust, a chonic case of which will lead to water and fire insufficiency. Water that cannot be stored will flood upward to be phlegm. It is a proper treatment to restrain fire so that water refrains from decending. When supplementing kidney, one must add medicinals extremely hot in property in order to have sufficient water to restrain fire, and sufficient fire to warm water as well. Only when fire and water are both harmonized, will water not flood to be phlegm. Formula:

熟地	shú dì	Prepared root of Rehmannia glutinosa	1 liang
山萸	shān yú	Fruit of Cornus officinalis	5 qian
肉桂	ròu guì	Bark of Cinnamonum cassia	2 qian
牛膝	niú xī	Root of Achyranthes bidentata	3 qian
五味子	wǔ wèi zǐ	Fruit of Schisandra chinensis	1 qian

The phlegm descends with the first dose and vanishes with the second dose.

中氣又中痰

中氣中痰，雖若中之異，而實中於氣之虛也。氣虛自然多痰，痰多必然耗氣，雖分而實合也。方用：

人參、甘草各壹兩，半夏、南星、茯苓各叁錢，附子壹錢，水煎服。

參原是氣分之神劑，而亦消痰之妙藥。半夏、南星，雖逐痰之神品，而亦扶氣之正藥。附子、甘草，一仁一勇，相濟而成。

Phlegm Syndrome and Qi4 Syndrome

Qi4 syndrome and phlegm syndrome, though seemingly different, are in fact both based on qi4 deficiency. Qi4 deficiency leads to excessive phlegm, which in turn consumes qi4. They are the same though apparently different. Formula:

人参	rén shēn	Root of Panax ginseng	1 liang
甘草	gān cǎo	Root of Glycyrrhiza uralensis	1 liang
半夏	bàn xià	Rhizome of Pinellia ternata	3 qian
南星	nán xīng	Rhioze of Pinallia	3 qian
茯苓	fú líng	Dried fungus of Poria cocos	3 qian
附子	fù zǐ	Lateral root of Aconitum carmichaeli	1 qian

Rén shēn is originally a divine medicinal for *qi4 aspect*[69], it is also an extremely effective medicinal for resolving phlegm. **Bàn xià** and **nán xīng**, though regarded as magic medicinals for dispelling phlegm, they are used to restore upright qi4 as well. **Fù zǐ** and **gān cǎo**, one is

[69] *qi4 aspect*: the second stratum of the body deeper than the defense aspect, often referring to the lung, gallbladder, spleen, stomach and large intestine.

benevolent and the other courageous, complement and coordinate each other.

濕嗽

秋傷於溼，若用烏梅粟殼等味，斷乎不效。方用：

陳皮、當歸、甘草、枳殼、桔梗各壹錢，白朮貳錢，水煎服。

三劑帖然矣。冬嗽皆秋傷於溼也，豈可拘於受寒乎。

Damp Phlegm

For patients damaged by dampness in autumn, the prescription of medicinals like **wū méi** and **yīng sù ké** is not at all effective. Formula:

陳皮	chén pí	Peel of Citrus reticulata	1 qian
當歸	dāng guī	Root of Angelica polimorpha	1 qian
甘草	gān cǎo	Root of Glycyrrhiza uralensis	1 qian
枳殼	zhǐ ké	Dried peel of Aurantii fructus	1 qian
桔梗	jié gěng	Root of Platycodon grandiflorum	1 qian
白朮	bái zhú	Rhizome of Atractylodes macrocephala	2 qian

Three packets of the midicinals will cure. Winter cough is always caused by damp damage during the autum. Why should we restrict therapy to cold affection?

久嗽

方用：

人參伍錢，益智仁伍分，白芍、棗仁各叁錢，五味子、白芥子各壹錢，水煎服。二劑後，服六味地黃丸。

方用：

瓜蔞仁去油，烏梅各伍錢，薄荷、甘草各伍分，人參童便浸、五味子酒蒸、寒水石火煅、杏仁、硼砂各壹錢，貝母叁兩，胡桃仁貳錢去油，蜜丸櫻桃大，淨綿包之，口中噙化。虛勞未曾失血，脈未數者，皆用之。無論老少神麴效，十粒見功，二十粒愈。又方用：

人參、當歸、細茶各一錢，水煎，連渣嚼盡，一、二劑即愈。

Chronic Cough

Formula:

人參	rén shēn	Root of Panax ginseng	5 qian
益智仁	yì zhì rén	Fruit of Sharpleaf Galangal	5 fen

白芍 bái sháo Root of Paeonia lactiflora 3 qian

棗仁 zǎo rén Seed of Ziziphus jujuba 3 qian

五味子 wǔ wèi zǐ Fruit of Schisandra chinensis 1 qian

白芥子 bái jiè zǐ Seed of Brassica alba 1 qian

After two doses, take *Liu Wei Di Huang* Pills.

Formula:

瓜蔞仁去油 guā lóu rén Seed of Trichosanthes Kirilowii (deoiled) 5 qian

烏梅 wū méi Unripe fruit of Prunus mume 5 qian

薄荷 bò hé Plant of Mentha Haplocalyx 5 fen

甘草 gān cǎo Root of Glycyrrhiza uralensis 5 fen

人參 rén shēn Root of Panax ginseng 1 qian (soaked in boy's urine)

五味子 wǔ wèi zǐ Fruit of Schisandra chinensis 1 qian (Steamed in wine)

寒水石 hán shuǐ shí Sodium calcium sulfate (forged) 1 qian

杏仁 xìng rén Dried seed of Prunus armeniaca 1 qian

硼砂 péng shà Borax 1 qian

貝母 bèi mǔ Bulb of Fritillaria cirrhosa 3 liang

胡桃仁 hú táo rén Walnut meat (deoiled) 2 qian

Make honeyed pills in size of cherry, wrap one pill up in a piece of clean cotton cloth, and hold the pack in mouth till dissolving. The formula is for consumptive disease without *loss of blood*[70] or rapid pulse. It is miraculously effective to both the young and the old. In ten pills the effect shows and in twenty pills the disease cures. Another formula:

人參	rén shēn	Root of Panax ginseng	1 qian
當歸	dāng guī	Root of Angelica polimorpha	1 qian
細茶	xì chá	Tea leaves	1 qian

For water decoction. The decoction is to be taken with chewing up the dregs. One or two doses will cure.

肺嗽兼補腎

肺嗽之證，本是肺虛，其補肺也明矣，奈何兼補腎乎？蓋肺經之氣，夜必歸於腎，若肺金為心火所傷，必求救於其子，子若力量不足，將何以救其母哉？方用：

熟地、麥冬各壹錢，紫苑伍分，山萸肆錢，元參伍錢，蘇子、牛膝各壹錢，沙參、天冬貳錢，水煎服。

---

[70] *loss of blood*: a general term for various kinds of profuse bleeding, the same as hemorrhage.

Lung Cough with Kidney Supplementation

Syndrome of lung cough originally is due to lung deficiency and it is obvious we should supplement the lung. Why is kidney concurrently supplemented? Because qi4 of lung meridian returns to kidney at night, and if the lung metal is hurt by heart fire, it seeks help from its child, but if the child's strength is insufficient, what does he rely on to save his mother? Formula:

熟地	shú dì	Prepared root of Rehmannia glutinosa	1 qian
麥冬	mài dōng	Tuber of Ophiopogon japonicus	1 qian
紫菀	zǐ wǎn	Root and rhizome of Aster tataricus	5 fen
山萸	shān yú	Fruit of Cornus officinalis	4 qian
元參	yuán shēn	Root of Scrophularia ningpoensis	5 qian
蘇子	sū zǐ	Seed of Perilla frutescens	1 qian
牛膝	niú xī	Root of Achyranthes bidentata	1 qian
沙參	shā shēn	Root of Adenophora tetraphylla	2 qian
天冬	tiān dōng	Tuber of Asparagus cochinchinensis	2 qian

喘證門

Chapter 6 Dyspnea

氣治法

氣虛氣實，不可不平之也。氣實者非氣實，乃正氣虛而邪氣實也。法當用補正之藥，而加祛逐之品，則正氣足而邪氣消矣。方用：人參、白朮、麻黃、半夏、甘草各壹錢，柴胡貳錢，白芍叁錢，水煎服。

推而廣之，治氣非一條也。氣陷，補中益氣湯可用；氣衰，六君子湯可採；氣寒，人參白朮附子湯可施；氣虛，則用四君子湯；氣鬱，則用歸脾湯；氣熱用生脈散；氣喘用獨參湯；氣動用二陳湯加人參；氣壅塞用射干湯；氣逆用逍遙散。

氣虛則羸弱，氣實則壯盛，氣虛用前方，實者另一方：白朮、柴胡、甘草、梔子各壹錢，茯苓叁錢，白芍貳錢，陳皮、枳殼各伍分，山查拾個，水煎服。

Qi Treatment Therapies

Qi4, whether deficient or excessive, should be leveled. The excess of qi4 is not upright qi4 in excess, but upright qi4 in deficiency and pathogenic qi4 in excess. It is a proper therapy to use upright-qi4 tonifying medicinals together with medicinals for elimination and dispersion, so that upright qi4 suffices and pathogens wane. Formula:

人參	rén shēn	Root of Panax ginseng	1 qian
白朮	bái zhú	Rhizome of Atractylodes macrocephala	1 qian
麻黃	má huáng	Stalk of Ephedra sinica	1 qian
半夏	bàn xià	Rhizome of Pinellia ternata	1 qian
甘草	gān cǎo	Root of Glycyrrhiza uralensis	1 qian
柴胡	chái hú	Root of Bupleurum chinense	2 qian
白芍	bái sháo	Root of Paconialactiflora Pall.	3 qian

In like manner, there is more than one way of qi4 treatment: *Bu Zhong Yi Qi4 Tang* for *qi4 fall*[71]; *Liu Jun Zi Tang* for qi4 debilitation; *Ren Shen Bai Shu Fu Zi Tang* for qi4 cold; *Si Jun Zi Tang* for qi4 deficiency; *Gui Pi Tang* for *qi4 movement stagnation*[72]; *Sheng Mai Powder* for qi4 heat;

[71] *qi4 fall*: a pathological change of deficient qi4 marked by failure in its lifting or holding function, also known as qi4 sinking.

[72] *qi4 movement stagnation*: depressed and stagnant flow of qi4 that causes dysfunction of internal organs and meridians/channels, the same as qi4 stagnation.

Du Shen Tang for shortness of breath; *Er Chen Tang* with **rén shēn** for qi4 wind; *Shen Gan Tang* for qi4 Blockage; *Xiao Yao San* for *qi4 counterflow*[73]. Qi4 deficiency induces frailness, and qi4 excess leads to sturdiness. The above formula treats qi4 deficiency. The following formula is for qi4 excess:

白朮 bái zhú Rhizome of Atractylodes macrocephala 1 qian
柴胡 chái hú Root of Bupleurum chinense 1 qian
甘草 gān cǎo Root of Glycyrrhiza uralensis 1 qian
梔子 zhī zǐ Fruit of Gardenia jasminoides 1
qian 茯苓 fú líng Dried fungus of Poria cocos 3 qian
白芍 bái sháo Root of Paconialactiflora Pall. 2 qian
陳皮 chén pí Dried Tangerine peel 5 fen
枳殼 zhǐ ké Prepared Slice of Fructus Aurantii 5 fen
山查 shān zhā Fruit of Crateagus pinnatifida 10 pcs.

氣喘

凡人氣喘而上者，人以為氣有餘也，殊不知氣盛當作氣虛看，有餘當作不足看，若認作肺氣之盛，而用蘇葉、

[73] *qi4 counterflow:* reversal of the normal downward flow of qi4.

桔梗、百部、豆根之類，去生遠矣。方用：

人參參兩，牛膝叁錢，熟地、麥冬各伍錢，山萸肆錢，胡桃參個，枸杞、五味子各壹錢，生薑伍片，水煎服。

此方不治肺，而正所以治肺也。或疑人參乃健脾土之藥，既宜補腎，不宜多用人參。不知腎水大虛，一時不能遽生，非急補其氣，則元陽一線，必且斷絕。況人參少用則泛上，多用即下行。妙在用人參三兩，使下達病原，補氣以生腎水。方中熟地、山萸之類，同氣相求，直入命門，又何患其多哉？若病重之人，尤宜多加。但喘有初起之喘，有久病之喘，初起之喘多實邪，久病之喘多氣虛，實邪喘者必抬肩，氣虛喘者微微氣息耳。此方治久病之喘，若初起之喘，四磨、四七湯，一劑即止喘，不獨肺氣虛而腎水竭也。

Shortness of Breath

Shortness of breath is often regarded as qi4 surplus, but it is rarely known that qi4 excess has been treated as qi4 deficiency, and the excess has been treated as deficiency. If taken as lung qi4 excess and treat with medicinals like **sū yè**, **jié gěng**, **bǎi bù** and **dòu gēn**, death befalls in no time. Formula:

人參	rén shēn	Root of Panax ginseng	3 liang
牛膝	niú xī	Root of Achyranthes bidentata	3 qian
熟地	shú dì	Prepared root of Rehmannia glutinosa	5 qian
麥冬	mài dōng	Tuber of Ophiopogon japonicus	5 qian
山萸	shān yú	Fruit of Cornus officinalis	4 qian
胡桃	hú táo	Walnut	1 pc.
枸杞	gǒu qǐ	Fruit of Lycium chinensis	1 qian
五味子	wǔ wèi zǐ	Fruit of Schisandra chinensis	1 qian
生薑	shēng jiāng	Fresh root of Zingiber officinale	5 slices

This formula treats lung by not treating lung (directly). People have doubts that **rén shēn** fortifies the spleen, but as for kidney tonification, **rén shēn** should not have been used in such a large dosage. They have no idea that kidney water is seriously deficient and (water) cannot be engendered in a short time span, then qi4 must be tonified urgently so that the trace of *source yang* 元陽 won't disappear. Moreover, efficacy of **rén shēn** floats upward if used in light dose, and it goes down if used in heavy dose. The genius of this formula consists in its use of three liang of **rén shēn**, efficacy of which goes down to the pathogens while tonifying qi4 to engender kidney water. Medicinals like **shú dì** and **shān yú** are of similar property and they both enter directly into the life gate. The heavy dosage is not a problem. The severe patients should be prescribed with a even larger quantity. However, shortness of breath is classified into onset shortness and prolonged shortness. The onset one is mostly of excess, while prolonged shortness is chiefly of qi4 deficiency. The former has symptoms of shoulder lifting, and the latter just gives short breath lightly. This formula is for prolonged shortness of breath. As for onset shortness, one dose of *Si Mo Tang*, or *Si Qi Tang* will cure, and there will not be any deterioration of lung qi4 deficiency and kidney water exhaustion.

實喘

方用：

黃芩貳錢，柴胡、甘草各伍分，麥冬叁錢，蘇葉、烏藥、半夏、山豆根各壹錢，水煎服。

一劑喘定，不必再劑也。凡實喘證，氣大急，喉中必作聲，肩必抬，似重而實輕也。

Dyspnea of Excess

Formula:

黄芩	huáng qín	Root of Baical Skullcap	2 qian
柴胡	chái hú	Root of Bupleurum chinense	5 fen
甘草	gān cǎo	Root of Glycyrrhiza uralensis	5 fen
麥冬	mài dōng	Tuber of Ophiopogon japonicus	3 qian
蘇葉	sū yè	Foliage of Perilla frutescens	1 qian
烏藥	wū yào	Root of Combined Spicebush	1 qian
半夏	bàn xià	Rhizome of Pinellia ternata	1 qian
山豆根	shān dòu gēn	Root of Menispermum dauricum DC.	1 qian

In one dose the shortness of breath will be gone and no more doses are needed. Dyspnea of excess has symptoms of short urgent breath, grunting in throat, shoulder lifting, which all looks like those of serious diseases though in fact a light one.

虛喘

大抵此等證，氣少息，喉無聲，肩不抬也。乃腎氣大虛，脾氣又復將絕，故奔沖而上，欲絕不絕也。方用救絕湯：人參、熟地各一兩，山萸三錢，牛膝、五味子、白芥子各一錢，麥冬五錢，水煎服。

Dyspnea of Deficiency

Dyspnea of deficiency[74] in most cases has symptoms of light breath but without throat sounds, and shoulder lifting. It is due to the utmost deficiency of kidney qi4 and the virtually extinguished spleen qi4 rushing upward. The formula is *Jiu Jue Tang* [pinyin: jiù jué tāng, 救絕湯, Emergent Rescue Decoction]:

人參	rén shēn	Root of Panax ginseng	1 liang
熟地	shú dì	Prepared root of Rehmannia glutinosa	1 liang
山萸	shān yú	Fruit of Cornus officinalis	3 qian
牛膝	niú xī	Root of Achyranthes bidentata	1 qian
五味子	wǔ wèi zǐ	Fruit of Schisandra chinensis	1 qian
白芥子	bái jiè zǐ	Seed of Brassica alba (L.) Boiss.	1 qian
麥冬	mài dōng	Tuber of Ophiopogon japonicus	5 qian

[74] *dyspnea of deficiency*: dyspnea due to insufficient lung and kidney qi, marked by shortness of breath and dyspnea upon exertion, usually gradual on onset and chronic in nature.

氣短似喘

此證似喘而非實喘也。若非實喘治之，立死。蓋氣短乃腎氣虛耗，氣沖上焦，壅塞於肺經，此不足之證也。方用：

人參二兩，熟地一兩，山萸、牛膝、補骨脂、枸杞各三錢，麥冬五錢，胡桃三個去皮，五味子二錢，水煎服。三劑氣平喘定。

此方妙在用人參之多，能下達氣原，挽回於無何有之鄉。又純是補肺補腎之品，子母相生，水氣自旺，則火氣自安於故宅，不上沖於喉門矣。

Dyspnea-like Shortness of Breath

This symptom is dyspnea-like, though not excessive dyspnea. If treated as dyspena of excess, death befalls in no time. The shortness of breath is caused by kidney qi4 deficiency and consumption, and qi4 rushes to the upper energizer and blocks lung meridian to induce breath difficulty, which is a symptom of deficiency. Formula:

人參	rén shēn	Root of Panax ginseng	2 liang
熟地	shú dì	Prepared root of Rehmannia glutinosa	1 liang

山萸	shān yú	Fruit of Cornus officinalis	3 qian
牛膝	niú xī	Root of Achyranthes bidentata	3 qian
補骨脂	bǔ gǔ zhī	Fruit of Malaytea Scurfpea	3 qian
枸杞	gǒu qǐ	Fruit of Lycium chinensis	3 qian
麥冬	mài dōng	Tuber of Ophiopogon japonicas	5 qian
胡桃	hú táo	Walnut	3 pcs. (without shell)
五味子	wǔ wèi zǐ	Fruit of Schisandra chinensis	2 qian

Three doses eliminate the shortness of breath. The beauty of this formula consists in its heavy dosage of **rén shēn**, efficacy of which goes down to the pathogens to cure the incurable. Moreover, the medicinals are purely for tonification of lung and kidney with mother-and-child reinforcement, so water and qi4 thrives all in their own rights and fire qi4 settles in its own abode, and will not rush upward to the gate of throat.

抬肩大喘

人忽感風邪，寒入於肺，以致喘息、肩抬、氣逆，痰吐不出，身不能臥。方用:

柴胡、茯苓、麥冬、桔梗各二錢，黃芩、當歸、甘草、半夏、射干各一錢，水煎服。

此方妙在用柴胡、射干、桔梗，以發舒肺金之氣，半夏以去痰，黃芩以去火。蓋感寒邪，內必變為熱證，故用黃芩以清解之。然徒用黃芩，雖曰清火，轉足以遏抑其火，而火未必伏也。有射干、桔梗、柴胡一派辛散之品，則足以消火滅邪矣。

Serious Dyspnea with Shoulder Lifting

When people contracts pathogenic wind, cold enters the lung and cause symptoms like heavy breath, shoulder lifting, qi4 *counterflow*[75], phlegm that cannot be spitted out and patients cannot lie down. Formula:

柴胡	chái hú	Root of Bupleurum chinense	2 qian
茯苓	fú líng	Dried fungus of Poria cocos	2 qian
麥冬	mài dōng	Tuber of Ophiopogon japonicus	2 qian
桔梗	jié gěng	Root of Platycodon grandiflorum	2 qian
黃芩	huáng qín	Root of Baical Skullcap	1 qian
當歸	dāng guī	Root of Angelica polimorpha	1 qian
甘草	gān cǎo	Root of Glycyrrhiza uralensis	1 qian
半夏	bàn xià	Rhizome of Pinellia ternata	1 qian

[75] *qi4 counterflow*: reversal of the normal downward flow of qi4.

射幹 shè gān Rhizome of Belamcanda chinensis 1 qian

The genius of this formula lies in its use of **chái hú**, **shè gān** and **jié gěng** to spread lung qi4, as well as in its use of **bàn xià** to dispel phlegm and **huáng qín** to eliminate fire. Once contracted with cold, patient will have internal heat, therefore **huáng qín** is used to clear away the heat. **Huáng qín** may inhibit heat from rampaging but it cannot control fire. The prescription of pungent-dispersing medicinals of **shè gān**, **jié gěng** and **chái hú** is enough to extinguish fire and eliminate pathogens.

腎寒氣喘

人有氣喘不能臥、吐痰如湧泉者，舌不燥而喘不止，一臥即喘，此非外感之寒邪，乃腎中之寒氣也。蓋腎中無火，則水無所養，乃泛上而為痰。方用：

六味地黃湯 加桂、附，大劑飲之，蓋人之臥，必腎氣與肺氣相安，而後河車之路平安而無奔越也。

Kidney-cold Dyspnea

Some patients of dyspnea cannot lie down, their spit is like a fountain, and their tongues are wet while the panting does not stop. Once lying down, they will pant. This is not an external contraction of cold, but cold qi4 of kidney. When there is no fire in kidney, water cannot be retained and will flood upward to form phlegm. The prescription is heavy dosage of *Liu Wei Di Huang Tang* with **fù zǐ** and **ròu guì**. When people lie down, kidney qi4 and lung qi4 must co-exit, then the pathway of waterwheel is safe and there is no rampant flooding.

腎火扶肝上沖

凡人腎火，逆扶肝氣而上沖，以致作喘，甚有吐紅粉痰者，此又腎火炎，上以燒肺金，肺熱不能剋肝，而龍雷之火升騰矣。方用：

沙參、地骨皮各壹兩，麥冬伍錢，丹皮叁錢，甘草叁分，桔梗伍分，白芍伍錢，白芥子貳錢，水煎服。

此方妙在地骨皮清骨中之火，沙參、丹皮以養陰，白芍平肝，麥冬清肺，甘草、桔梗引入肺經，則痰消而喘定矣。

Kidney Fire Rushes upwards Coercing Liver

Kidney fire may rush upwards coercing liver qi4 to induce dyspnea. A deteriorated case is the symptom of pink-colored phlegm. This is caused by lung metal, as burned by the kidney fire flaming, turns hot and cannot restrain liver, so that the fire rushes upwards rampantly. Formula:

沙参	shā shēn	Root of Adenophora tetraphylla	1 liang
地骨皮	dì gǔ pí	Root bark of Lycium chinense Mill.	1 liang
麥冬	mài dōng	Tuber of Ophiopogon japonicus	5 qian
丹皮	dān pí	Root bark of Paeonia suffruticosa Andr.	3 qian
甘草	gān cǎo	Root of Glycyrrhiza uralensis	3 fen
桔梗	jié gěng	Root of Platycodon grandiflorum	5 fen
白芍	bái sháo	Root of Paconialactiflora Pall.	5 qian
白芥子	bái jiè zǐ	Seed of Brassica alba (L.) Boiss.	2 qian

The genius of this formula consists in its use of **dì gǔ pí** which clears away fire, **shā shēn** and **dān pí** which tonifies yin, **bái sháo** which pacifies liver, **mài dōng** which clears away lung heat, and **gān cǎo** and **jié gěng** which channel efficacy of the medicinals into lung meridian, so that phlegm is eliminated and dyspnea settled.

假熱氣喘吐痰

人有假熱氣喘吐痰者，人以為熱而非熱也，乃下元寒極，逼其火而上喘也。此最危急之證，苟不急救其腎水與命門之火，則一線之微，必然斷絕。方用：

熟地肆兩，山藥、麥冬各參兩，五味子、牛膝各壹兩，附子，肉桂各壹錢，水煎冷服。一劑而愈。

False-heat Dyspnea and Phlegm

The syndrome of false-heart dyspnea and phlegm may be mistaken for true heat. The dyspnea is caused by extreme cold of kidney qi4 which forces the fire to flame upward. This is one of the most perilous diseases, and if kidney water and life gate fire is not tonified urgently, the trace of life will be gone. Formula:

熟地	shú dì	Prepared root of Rehmannia glutinosa	4 liang
山藥	shān yào	Root stock of Dioscorea opposite	1 liang
麥冬	mài dōng	Tuber of Ophiopogon japonicus	1 liang
五味子	wǔ wèi zǐ	Fruit of Schisandra chinensis	1 liang
牛膝	niú xī	Root of Achyranthes bidentata	1 liang
附子	fù zǐ	Lateral root of Aconitum carmichaeli	1 qian

肉桂 ròu guì	Bark of Cinnamomum cassia	1 qian

The decoction shall be taken cold, and one dose will cure.

喘嗽

人有喘而且嗽者，人以為氣虛而有風痰也，誰知是氣虛不能歸源於腎，而肝木挾之作祟乎。法當峻補其腎，少助以引火之品，則氣自歸源於腎，而喘嗽俱止。方用：

人參壹兩，熟地貳兩，麥冬伍錢，茯苓叁錢，牛膝、枸杞、白朮、五味子、兔絲子各壹錢，水煎服。連服五劑，必有大功。倘以四磨、四七湯治之，則不效矣。

Panting Cough

Panting cough may often be regarded as *wind phlegm*[76] due to qi4-deficiency. It is rarely known that qi4 deficiency should not be attributed to kidney, but to liver wood which is held under duress. Proper treatment is urgent tonification of kidney assisted by fire-lighting medicinals, so that qi4 returns to kidney in its own rights and panting cough stops. Formula:

[76] *wind phlegm*: a combined pathogen of wind and phlegm.

人參	rén shēn	Root of Panax ginseng	1 liang
熟地	shú dì	Prepared root of Rehmannia glutinosa	2 liang
麥冬	mài dōng	Tuber of Ophiopogon japonicas	qian
茯苓	fú líng	Dried fungus of Poria cocos	3 qian
牛膝	niú xī	Root of Achyranthes bidentata	1 qian
枸杞	gǒu qǐ	Fruit of Lycium chinensis	1 qian
白朮	bái zhú	Rhizome of Atractylodes macrocephala	1 qian
五味子	wǔ wèi zǐ	Fruit of Schisandra chinensis	1 qian
菟絲子	tù sī zǐ	Seed of Cuscuta chinensis	1 qian

Five dosages taken successively will bring about great success which would have been impossible if *Si Mo Tang* or *Si Qi Tang* were used.

貞元飲

此方專治喘而脈微濇者。

熟地參兩，當歸柒錢，甘草壹錢，水煎服。婦人多此證。

Zhen Yuan Cold Decoction

This is a specific formula for those who pant with slightly unsmooth pulse:

熟地	shú dì	Prepared root of Rehmannia glutinosa	3 liang
當歸	dāng guī	Root of Angelica polimorpha	7 qian
甘草	gān cǎo	Root of Glycyrrhiza uralensis	1 qian

Women often have this syndrome.

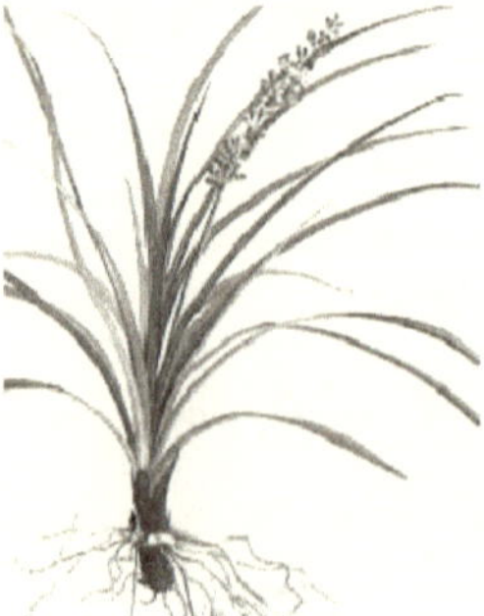

吐血門

Chapter 7 Hematemesis

陽證吐血

人有感暑傷氣，忽然吐血盈盆，人以為陰虛也，不知陰虛吐血與陽虛不同。陰虛吐血，人安靜無躁動；陽虛必大熱作渴，欲飲冷水，舌必有刺；陰虛口不渴而舌胎滑也。法當清胃火，不必止血也。方用：

人參、當歸、香薷、石膏各叁錢，荊芥壹錢，青蒿伍錢，水煎服。

此方乃陽證吐血之神麴劑也。方中雖有解暑之品，然補正多於解暑，去香薷一味，實可同治。但此方衹可用一、二劑，即改六味地黃湯。

Yang Disease Blood Ejection[77]

People, who have contracted summerheat with qi4 damage, may eject blood all of sudden in a large quantity. Believed as yin deficiency, it is in fact yin-deficiency blood ejection which is different from the yang-deficiency one.

[77] *Blood ejection:* Blood ejection is called Hematemesis in modern language. (or something like this)

Patients of the former are peaceful with no sign of restlessness; while those of the latter will have thirst caused by great heat, a yearning for cold water, and a prickly tongue. The yin-deficiency patients have no thirst, but a *slippery coating*[78]on their tongue. It is proper to clear stomach fire, rather than to stop bleeding. Formula:

人參	rén shēn	Root of Panax ginseng	3 qian
當歸	dāng guī	Root of Angelica polimorpha	3 qian
香薷	xiāng rú	Herb of Haichow Elsholtzi	3 qian
石膏	shí gāo	Gypsum	3 qian
荊芥	jīng jiè	Leaf of Schizonepeta tenuifolia	1 qian
青蒿	qīng hāo	Foliage of Artemisiae Apiacceae	5 qian

This is a sovereign remedy for yang symptom blood ejection. Although there are some medicinals which release summerheat in this formula, there are more medicinals supplemeningt the right qi4. This formula is also effective if without **xiāng rú.** However, it can only be prescribed for

[78] *slippery coating*: a moist tongue coating with excessive fluid, feels slippery.

one or two doses before changing to Liuwei Dihuang Tang (六味地黄湯).

大怒吐血

其吐也，或傾盆而出，或沖口而來，一時昏暈，死在頃刻。以止血治之，則氣悶不安；以補血治之，則胸滿不受；有變證蜂起而死者，不可不治之得法也。方用解血平氣湯：

白芍、當歸各貳兩，炒荊芥、黑梔各叁錢，紅花貳錢，柴胡捌分，甘草壹錢，水煎服。

一劑而氣平舒，二劑而血止息，三劑而病大愈。

此證蓋怒傷肝，不能平其氣，以致吐血。若不先舒其氣，而遽止血，則愈激動肝火之氣，必氣愈旺而血愈吐矣。方中用白芍平肝又舒氣，荊芥、柴胡引血歸經，當歸、紅花，生新去舊，安有不愈者哉？

Blood Ejection due to Rage

When blood is ejected either in large quantities or in a sudden outburst with patients' fainting, death befalls in no time. If to stop bleeding, the patient will feel stuffy and restless. If to supplement blood, the patient will feel fullness and rigidity in their chest. These symptoms, if not properly treated, may have swarms of deterioration. Formula: Jie Xue Ping Qi4 Tang [pinyin: jiě xuè píng qì tāng, 解血平氣湯, The Decoction for Cleasing Blood and Normalizing Qi4]:

白芍	bái sháo	Root of Paeonia lactiflora	2 liang
當歸	dāng guī	Root of Angelica polimorpha	2 liang
炒荊芥	chǎo jīng jiè	Fried leaf of Schizonepeta tenuifolia	3 qian
黑梔	hēi zhì	Fruit or root of Gardenia stenphylla Merr.	3 qian
紅花	hóng huā	Safflower	2 qian
柴胡	chái hú	Root of Bupleurum chinense	8 fen
甘草	gān cǎo	Root of Glycyrrhiza uralensis	1 qian

The first dose soothes and normalizes qi4, the second dose stops bleeding, and the third one substantially heals.

Anger damages liver and if qi4 circulation is abnormal, blood ejection forms. If qi4 is not soothed before blood stopping, qi4 of liver fire will be stirred even more. The more effulgent the qi4 is, the more blood will be ejected. This formula uses **bái sháo** to calm liver and soothe qi4, **jīng jiè** and **chái hú** to guide blood into meridians, **dāng guī** and

hóng huā to do away with the old and promote generation. How could it fail?

吐血

此證人非以為火盛，即以陰虧。用涼藥以瀉火，乃火愈退而血愈多；用滋陰之味，止血之品仍不效，誰知是血不歸經乎？治法當用補氣之藥，而佐以引血歸經之味，不止血而血自止矣。方用：

人參伍錢，當歸壹兩，丹皮炒、黑芥穗各叁錢，水煎服，一劑而止。

此方妙在不專補血，而反去補氣以補血，尤妙在不去止血，而去行血以止血。蓋血逢寒則凝，逢散則歸經，救死於呼吸之際，大有神功。

大凡吐血，多係不歸經之血。因何腑何藏而發，腑藏之血，吐則立死，此自然之理也。

Blood Ejection

People believe this syndrome is either due to fire exuberance or to yin deficiency. If cold medicinals are used to purge fire, the further the fire retreats, the more the blood bleeds. It is not effective either to use medicinals for yin tonification or blood stopping. They do not know it is that the *blood fails to stay in the meridian* [79]. Proper therapy is to supplement qi4 with assistance of medicinals that conduct blood into the meridians. The bleeding will then stop in its own rights. Formula:

人參	rén shēn	Root of Panax ginseng	5 qian
當歸	dāng guī	Root of Angelica polimorpha	1 liang
丹皮	dān pí	Bark of the root of Paeonia suffruticosa(fried)	3 qian
黑芥穗	hēi jiè suì	Carbionized Leaf of Schizonepetae	3 qian

One dose of decoction is enough.

The genius of this formula lies in that it does not supplement blood, but supplements qi4 in order to supplement blood. It is particularly ingenious in that it does not stop bleeding, but rather moves the blood, which is vital because blood congeals when cold and dissipates after entering the meridians. A life at stake is saved here. What a

[79] *blood failing to stay in the meridians*: a pathological change that causes extravasation of blood.

miraculous formula!

Blood ejection in most cases is due to blood's failure to stay in the meridians. It is sure that whether from any viscera or any bowel, blood, if ejected, may lead to instant death.

吐白血

血未有不紅者，何以名白血？不知久病之人，吐痰皆白沫，乃白血也。白沫何以名白血？以其狀似蟹涎，無敗痰存其中，實血而非痰也。若將所吐白沫露於星光之下，一夜必變紅矣。此沫出於腎，而腎火沸騰於咽喉，不得不吐者也。雖是白沫，而實腎中之精，豈特血而已哉？苟不速治，則白沫變為綠痰，無可如何矣。方用：

熟地、麥冬各壹兩，山藥、山萸、茯苓各伍錢，丹皮、澤瀉各貳錢，五味子壹錢，水煎，日日服之。

Ejection of White Blood

Blood is red in color, how come the name "white blood"? It is rarely known that patients of chronic diseases spit white foam named as "white blood". Why is it named like this? It is in a shape of crab dribble but without deteriorated phlegm in it, which is actually blood rather than phlegm. If exposed to star light, the foam turns red over night. The foam originates in kidney and is forced out of throat by the blazing of kidney fire. While in shape of white foam, it is in fact essence of kidney, not merely blood. If not treated duly, it will turn into a kind of greenish phlegm, which is incurable at all. Formula:

熟地	shú dì	Prepared root of Rehmannia glutinosa	1 liang
麥冬	mài dōng	Tuber of Ophiopogon japonicus	1 liang
山藥	shān yào	Root of Dioscorea opposita	5 qian
山萸	shān yú	Fruit of Cornus officinalis	5 qian
茯苓	fú líng	Dried fungus of Poria cocos	5 qian
丹皮	dān pí	Bark of the root of Paeonia suffruticosa	2 qian
澤瀉	zé xiè	Rhizome of Alisma plantago-aquatica	2 qian
五味子	wǔ wèi zǐ	Fruit of Schisandra chinensis	1 qian

Water decoction, to be taken once daily.

血不歸經

凡人血不歸經，或上或下，或四肢毛竅各處出血。循行經絡，外行於皮毛，中行於臟腑，內行於筋骨，上行於頭目兩手，下行於二便，一劑周身無非血路。一不歸經，斯各處妄行，有孔則鑽，有洞則洩，甚則嘔吐。或見於皮毛，或出於齒縫，或滲於臍腹，或露於二便，皆宜順其性以引之歸經。方用：

熟地、生地各五錢，當歸、白芍、麥冬各叁錢，荊芥、川芎、甘草、茜草根各一錢，水煎服。

此方即四物湯加減，妙在用茜草引血歸經。

Blood Failing to Stay in Meridians

When blood fails to stay in the meridians, it goes either upward and downward or to the extremities and body hair openings, causing bleeding everywhere. As to its circulation along the meridians and collaterals, its exterior movement covers the body hair and skin; It moves midway over the bowels and viscera and interiorly through the sinews and bones; It goes upward to the head and hands, downward to the lower orifices, causing bleeding all the way over human body. If blood fails to stay in meridians, it randomly flows, penetrates, leaks and even leads to ejection. It is shown on skin and body hair, through the teeth, out of umbilical abdomen or seen in urine and stool. It is a proper treatment to conform to its property and conduct it into the meridians. Formula:

熟地	shú dì	Prepared root of Rehmannia glutinosa	5 qian
生地	shēng dì	Fresh root of Rehmannia glutinosa	5 qian
當歸	dāng guī	Root of Angelica polimorpha	3 qian
白芍	bái sháo	Root of Paeonia lactiflora	3 qian
麥冬	mài dōng	Tuber of Ophiopogon japonicus	3 qian
荊芥	jīng jiè	Leaf of Schizonepeta tenuifolia	1 qian
川芎	chuān xiōng	Root of Ligusticum wallichii	1 qian
甘草	gān cǎo	Root of Glycyrrhiza uralensis	1 qian
茜草根	qiàn cǎo gen□	Root of Rubia Cordifolia	1 qian

This is an adjusted formula of *Si Wu Tang* [pinyin: sì wù tāng, 四物湯, Four-medicinal Decoction]. The beauty of this formula consists in its use of **qiàn cǎo** to conduct blood into the original meridians.

附三黑神麴奇散

丹皮炒黑七分，黑梔五分，真蒲黃炒黑一錢二分，川芎酒洗、貝母各一錢，生地酒洗一錢，水二樽，童便、藕汁各半樽，煎服。

此方治吐血神效無比，二劑止。六味地黃湯加麥冬、五味子，最能補腎滋肝。木得其養，則血有可藏之經而不外洩，血證最宜服之。

Attachment: San Hei Shen Qu Magic Powder

丹皮 dān pí Bark of the root of Paeonia suffruticosa 7 fen (fried to dark color)

黑梔 hēi zhì Fruit or root of Gardenia stenphylla Merr. 5 fen

真蒲黃 zhēn pú huáng Prepared pollen of Typha angustata 1 qian and 7 fen (fried to dark color)

川芎 chuān xiōng Root of Ligusticum wallichii 1 qian (washed in liquor)

貝母 bèi mǔ Bulb of Fritillaria cirrhosa 1 qian

生地 shēng dì Fresh root Rehmannia glutinosa 1 qian (washed in liquor)

To be decocted in two containers of water with half container of **tóng biàn** (boy's urine) and another half container of lotus root juice.

This is a magic formula for blood ejection, and in two doses the ejection will stop. *Liu Wei Di Huang Tang* added with **mài dōng** and **wǔ wèi zǐ** best tonifies kidney and moistens liver. Once liver wood is raised, blood will be hoarded in its meridians and will not leak. This formula is most applicable to blood syndromes.

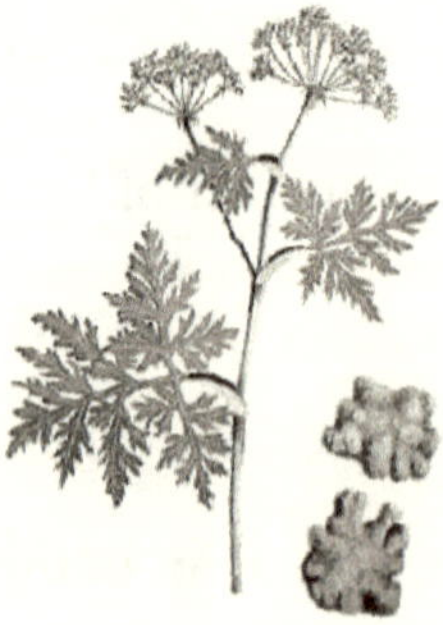

嘔吐門

Chapter 8 Vomiting

脾胃證辨

人有能食而不能化者，乃胃不病而脾病也，當補脾。而補脾尤宜補腎中之火，蓋腎火能生脾土也。不能食，食之而安然者，乃脾不病而胃病也，不可補腎中之火，當補心火，蓋心火能生胃土也。世人一見不飲食，動曰脾胃虛也，殊不知胃之虛寒責之心，脾之虛寒責之腎也，不可不辨也。

Spleen and Stomach Syndrome Differentiation

Those who can eat but cannot digest properly have a spleen disease instead of a stomach one. Proper treatment is to tonify spleen, and it is more appropriate to tonify kidney fire which can engender spleen earth. Those who cannot eat but feel much better after food intake have a stomach disease instead of a spleen one. This shall be treated with tonifying heart fire rather than kidney fire, because the heart fire generates stomach earth. Common people think it is spleen-stomach weakness once they eat less, but they do not know the heart is responsible for the *deficiency cold*[80] of stomach, while kidney is responsible for the deficiency cold of spleen. This must be differentiated.

反胃大吐

大吐之證，舌有芒刺，雙目紅腫，人以為熱也，誰知是腎水之虧乎？蓋脾胃必借腎水而滋潤，腎水一虧，致脾胃之火，沸騰而上，以致目紅腫而舌芒刺也。但此證時躁時靜，時欲飲水，及水到又不欲飲，即強之飲亦不甚快。此乃上假熱而下真寒也，宜六味地黃湯加桂、附，水煎服。

外治法：先以手擦其足心，使之極熱，然後用附子壹箇煎湯，用鵝翎掃之，隨乾隨掃，少頃即不吐矣。後以六味地黃湯，大劑飲之，即安然也。或逍遙散加黃連，亦立止也。無如世醫以雜藥投之而成噎嗝矣。方用：

熟地貳兩，山萸、元參各壹兩，當歸伍錢，五味子貳錢，牛膝、白芥子各叁錢，水煎服。蓋腎水不足，則大腸必乾而細，飲食入胃，難於下行，故反而上吐矣。

[80] *deficiency cold*: a pathological change arising when yang qi becomes insufficient and fails to provide adequate warmth.

Serious *Stomach Reflux*[81] Vomit

Patient with serious vomit have *prickly tongue*[82], swollen and red eyes. People think it is duo to heat though in fact due to kidney water deficiency. Spleen-stomach is nourished and moistened by kidney water. Under the circumstance of depletion of kidney water, spleen-stomach fire blazes upwards to induce prickly tongue together with swollen and red eyes. However, patients with this symptom fluctuates between agitation and quietness, sometimes patient wants to drink but refuse to drink when water is available, or drinks slowly even when he forces himself to, this is the false upper heat and true lower cold. Proper treatment is *Liu Wei Di Huang Tang* 六味地黄湯 added with **fù zǐ** and **ròu guì**.

For external treatment, rub patient's soles with both hands to make them extremely hot, then decoct one piece of **fù zǐ** and apply the decoction to his soles with a goose quill, repeat the application after the decoction dries and the patient's vomit will stop soon. A large dose of *Liu Wei Di*

---

81 *stomach reflux*: flowing back of the stomach contents into esophagus and mouth long after eating, also known as gastro esophageal reflux.

82 *prickly tongue*: a tongue with thorn-like protrusions on its surface.

Huang Tang 六味地黃湯 is then administered and the disease is cured. Another option is *Xiao Yao San* [pinyin: xiāo yáo sǎn, 逍遙散, Free and Easy Powder] with **huáng lián**, which stops the vomit instantly. However, common practitioners administer assorted medicines which may cause hiccup. Formula:

熟地	shú dì	Prepared root of Rehmannia glutinosa	2 liang
山萸	shān yú	Fruit of Cornus officinalis	1 liang
元參	yuán shēn	Root of Scrophularia ningpoensis	1 liang
當歸	dāng guī	Root of Angelica polimorpha	5 qian
五味子	wǔ wèi zǐ	Fruit of Schisandra chinensis	2 qian
牛膝	niú xī	Root of Achyranthes bidentata	3 qian
白芥子	bái jiè zǐ	Seed of Brassica alba	3 qian

Insufficiency of kidney water leads to dry and thin large intestines, food intake cannot descend but to turn upward.

寒邪犯腎大吐

寒入腎宮，將脾胃之水，挾之盡出，手足厥逆，小腹痛不可忍，以熱物熨之少快，否則寒冷難支，人多以為胃病，其實腎病也，方用：

附子壹箇、白朮肆兩、肉桂壹錢、乾薑叁錢、人參參兩，水煎服。

此藥下喉，便覺吐定，煎渣再服，安然如故。

Serious Vomit due to Cold-invaded Kidney

Cold penetrates into kidney, coerces and takes out spleen-stomach water. Patient has reversal cold of extremities and is unbearable pain in his lower abdomen, but somewhat relieved if a hot object is held against his lower abdomen, otherwise the cold is intolerable. Most people think it is a stomach complaint, though in fact a kidney one. Formula:

附子	fù zǐ	Lateral root of Aconitum carmichaeli	1 pc.
白朮	bái zhú	Rhizome of Atractylodes macrocephala	4 liang
肉桂	ròu guì	Bark of Cinnamonum cassia	1 qian
乾薑	gān jiāng	Dried root of Zingiber officinale	3 qian
人參	rén shēn	Root of Panax ginseng	3 liang

Once decoction goes down the throat, vomit quiets and the next decoction of the dregs cures.

嘔吐

世人皆以嘔吐為胃虛，誰知由於腎虛乎！故治吐不效，為窺見病之根也，方用：

人參、芡實各叁錢、白朮、薏仁各伍錢、砂仁伍粒、吳萸伍分，水煎服。

Vomit

People think that vomit is due to stomach deficiency, but rarely do they know that it is for kidney deficiency. Vomit is therefore not effectively treated because the root is not detected. Formula:

人參	rén shēn	Root of Panax ginseng	3 qian
芡實	qiàn shí□	Seed of Gordon Euryale	3 qian
白朮	bái zhú	Rhizome of Atractylodes macrocephala	5 qian
薏仁	yì rén	Seed kernel of Coix lachryma-jobi	5 qian
砂仁	shā rén	Fruit of Amomum villosum	5 pcs.
吳萸	wú yú	Leaf of Trichotomous Evodia	5 fen

火吐

此症若降火，則火由脾而入於大腸，必變為便血之症，法宜清火止吐，方用：

茯苓壹兩、人參貳錢、砂仁伍粒、黄連叁錢，水煎服。

Fire Vomit

If borne down, fire enters the large intestine through spleen and generates hematochezia. Proper treatment is to clear away fire to stop vomit. Formula:

茯苓	fú líng	Dried fungus of Poria cocos	1 liang
人參	rén shēn	Root of Panax ginseng	2 qian
砂仁	shā rén	Fruit of Amomum villosum	5 pcs.
黄連	huáng lián	Rhizome of Coptis chinensis	3 qian

寒吐

此症若降寒，則又引入腎而流於膀胱，必變為遺尿之症，法宜散寒止吐，方用：

白朮貳兩、人參伍錢、附子、乾薑各壹錢、丁香伍分，水煎服。

此方散寒而用補脾之品，則寒不能上越，而亦不得下行，勢不能不從臍出也。

Cold Vomit

Once borne down, cold is conducted into kidney and flows into bladder, which invariably results in *enuresis*[83]. Proper treatment is to dissipate cold to stop vomit. Formula:

白朮	bái zhú	Rhizome of Atractylodes macrocephala	2 liang
人參	rén shēn	Root of Panax ginseng	5 qian
附子	fù zǐ	Lateral root of Aconitum carmichaeli	1 qian
乾薑	gān jiāng	Dried root of Zingiber officinale	1 qian
丁香	dīng xiāng	Flower bud of Syzygium aromaticum	5 fen

This formula dissipates cold while tonifying spleen, so that the cold can neither float upward nor go down, but has to exit from the umbilicus.

胃吐

此症由於脾虛，脾氣不得下行，自必上反而吐，補脾則胃安，方用：

人參、茯苓各叁錢、白朮伍錢、甘草、肉桂、神麴、半夏各壹錢、砂仁參粒，水煎服。

此方治胃病，以補脾者何也？蓋胃為脾之關，關門之

[83] *enuresis*: involuntary discharge of urine during sleep.

沸騰，由於關中之潰亂，欲使關外之安靜，必先使關中之安寧，況方中砂仁半夏神麴等味，全是止吐之品，有不奏功者乎，此脾胃兩補之法也。

Stomach Vomit

The symptom is caused by spleen deficiency. Spleen qi4 cannot descend and in turn refluxes to cause vomit. The stomach will be tranquilized if spleen is tonified. Formula:

人參	rén shēn	Root of Panax ginseng	3 qian
茯苓	fú líng	Dried fungus of Poria cocos	3 qian
白朮	bái zhú	Rhizome of Atractylodes macrocephala	5 qian
甘草	gān cǎo	Root of Glycyrrhiza uralensis	1 qian
肉桂	ròu guì	Bark of Cinnamonum cassia	1 qian
神麴	shén qū	Medicated leaven	1 qian
半夏	bàn xià	Rhizome of Pinellia ternata	1 qian
砂仁	shā rén	Fruit of Amomum villosum	3 pcs.

Why is stomach treated through spleen tonification in this formula? Because stomach is the pass to spleen, and disorder out of the pass is caused by derangement within. To tranquilize the pass, spleen must be calmed first. Moreover, medicinals like **shā rén**, **bàn xià**, and **shén qū** of the formula are all for vomit stopping, how can the formula fail? This is the dual tonification of both spleen and stomach.

反胃

人有食入而即出者，乃腎水虛不能潤喉，故喉燥而即出也，方用：

熟地貳兩、山萸、茯苓、麥冬各伍錢、山藥壹兩、澤瀉、丹皮各叁錢、五味子貳錢，水煎服。

此症又有食久而反出者，乃腎火虛不能溫脾，故脾寒而反出也，方用 ：

熟地貳兩、山萸壹兩、山藥陸錢、澤瀉貳錢、茯苓、丹皮、附子、肉桂各叁錢，水煎服。（此即八味地黃，也可用生地桂枝）。

Stomach Reflux

Food, upon intake, is vomited up. This symptom is caused by a dry throat due to kidney water deficienty which renders moistening of the throat impossible. Formula:

熟地 shú dì Prepared root of Rehmannia glutinosa 2 liang

山萸 shān yú Fruit of Cornus officinalis 5 qian

茯苓 fú líng Dried fungus of Poria cocos 5 qian

麥冬 mài dōng Tuber of Ophiopogon japonicus 5 qian

山藥 shān yào Root of Dioscorea opposita 1 liang

澤瀉 zé xiè Rhizome of Alisma plantago-aquatica 3 qian

丹皮 dān pí Bark of the root of Paeonia suffruticosa 3 qian

五味子 wǔ wèi zǐ Fruit of Schisandra chinensis 2 qian

Another symptom is that long-taken food is vomited up, which a reflux due to spleen cold that is caused by the kidney fire deficiency which cannot warm the spleen. Formula:

熟地 shú dì Prepared root of Rehmannia glutinosa 2 liang

山萸 shān yú Fruit of Cornus officinalis 1 liang

山藥 shān yào Root of Dioscorea opposita 6 qian

澤瀉 zé xiè Rhizome of Alisma plantago-aquatica 2 qian

茯苓 fú líng Dried fungus of Poria cocos 3 qian

丹皮 dān pí Bark of the root of Paeonia suffruticosa 3 qian

附子 fù zǐ Lateral root of Aconitum carmichaeli 3 qian

肉桂 ròu guì Bark of Cinnamonum cassia 3 qian

(This is the *Ba Wei Di Huang* 八味地黃, we may as well use **shēng dì** and **guì zhī**).

胃寒

心腎兼補，治脾胃兩虛者固效，若單胃之虛寒，自宜獨治心之為妙，方用：

人參、遠志各壹兩、白朮、茯苓、蓮子、白芍各參兩、菖蒲、良薑、棗仁各伍錢、半夏、附子、白芥子各叁錢、山藥肆錢，蜜丸，每日白水送下五錢。

Stomach Cold

Dual tonification of both heart and kidney surely works for the dual deficiency of spleen and stomach. However, if there is only *deficiency cold*[84] of stomach, the proper solution is to treat heart alone. Formula:

人參	rén shēn	Root of Panax ginseng	1 liang
遠志	yuǎn zhì	Root of Polygala tenuifolia	1 liang
白朮	bái zhú	Rhizome of Atractylodes macrocephala	2 liang

[84] *deficiency cold*: a pathological change arising when yang qi becomes insufficient and fails to provide adequate warmth.

茯苓	fú líng	Dried fungus of Poria cocos	2 liang
蓮子	lián zǐ	Lotus seed	3 liang
白芍	bái sháo	Root of Paeonia lactiflora	3 liang
菖蒲	chāng pú	Rhizome of Acorus gramineus	5 qian
良薑	liáng jiāng	Rhizome of Alpinia officinarum Hance	5 qian
棗仁	zǎo rén	Seed of Ziziphus jujuba	5 qian
半夏	bàn xià	Rhizome of Pinellia ternata	3 qian
附子	fù zǐ	Lateral root of Aconitum carmichaeli	3 qian
白芥子	bái jiè zǐ	Seed of Brassica alba	3 qian
山藥	shān yào	Root of Dioscorea opposita	4 qian

Daily dose of five qian of honeyed pills, to be taken with boiled water.

腎寒吐瀉心寒胃弱

此症由於心寒胃弱，嘔吐不已，食久而出是也，下痢不止，五更時痛瀉三五次者是也，人以為脾胃之寒，服脾胃之藥而不效者何也，蓋胃為腎之關，而脾為腎之海，胃氣弱，不補命門之火，則心包寒甚，何以生胃土而消穀食，脾氣弱不補命門之火，則下焦虛冷，何以化飲食而生精華，故補脾胃，莫急於補腎也。方用：

熟地、茯苓、人参各參兩、山萸貳兩、山藥肆兩、附子、肉桂、五味子各壹兩、吳萸伍錢，蜜丸，每日空心白水送下五錢。

Kidney-cold Vomit & Diarrhea with Heart-cold Stomach Deficiency

This syndrome has symtpoms of heart-cold and stomach weakness, incessant vomit, reflux of long-taken food, constant *dysentery*[85], and diarrhea with stool in deep night. Normally considered as spleen-stomach cold, it is treated with medicinals for spleen-stomach diseases but with no avail. The reason is that stomach is the pass to kidney, while spleen is the sea of kidney. When kidney qi4 is weak, heart is extremely cold if the *life gate fire*[86] is not tonified. How can stomach earth be engendered to digest food? If life-gate fire is not tonified when spleen qi4 is weak, the lower energizer will be cold and deficient, how to digest food and generate essence? Therefore, spleen and stomach are tonified instead of a hurried tonification of the kidney. Formula:

---

[85] *dysentery*: a disease characterized by abdominal pain, tenesmus, diarrhea with stool containing mucus and blood

[86] *life gate fire*: innate fire from the life gate, a synonym of kidney yang.

熟地	shú dì	Prepared root of Rehmannia glutinosa	1 liang
茯苓	fú líng	Dried fungus of Poria cocos	1 liang
人參	rén shēn	Root of Panax ginseng	1 liang
山萸	shān yú	Fruit of Cornus officinalis	2 liang
山藥	shān yào	Root of Dioscorea opposita	4 liang
附子	fù zǐ	Lateral root of Aconitum carmichaeli	1 liang
肉桂	ròu guì	Bark of Cinnamonum cassia	1 liang
五味子	wǔ wèi zǐ	Fruit of Schisandra chinensis	1 liang
吳萸	wú yú	Leaf of Trichotomous Evodia	5 qian

Honeyed pills, daily dose of five qian is to be taken with boiled water when stomach is empty.

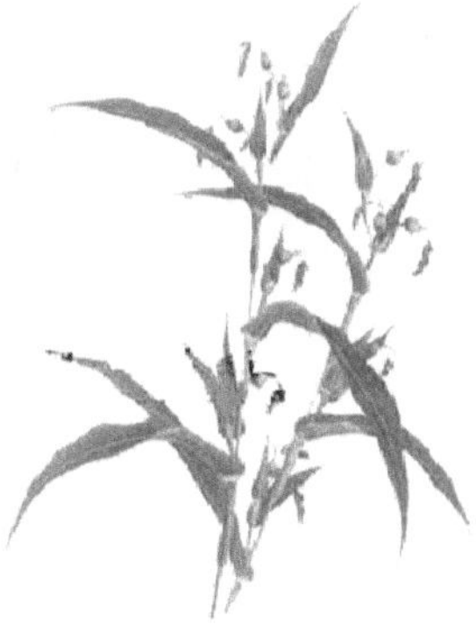

臌證門

Chapter 9 Tympanites

水臌

此證滿身皆水，按之如泥者是。若不急治，水流四肢，不得從膀胱出，則為死證矣。方用決流湯：

黑丑、甘草各貳錢，肉桂參分，車前壹兩，水煎服。

一劑水流斗餘，二劑全愈。斷勿與三劑也，與三劑反殺之矣。蓋二丑、甘遂，最善利水，又加肉桂、車前子，引火以入膀胱，利水而不走氣，不使牛、遂之過猛也。二劑之後，須改五苓散，調理二劑；再用六君子湯補脾可也；忌食鹽，犯之則不救矣。

諸臌證最忌寬中市醫多用五皮飲，描頭畫角，百無一效。

Ascites

Ascites is symptomized by accumulation of fluid all over patient's body which is sludge-like if pressed. If not promptly treated, fluid flows to the extremities instead of exiting from the bladder, and death befalls. The formula is

Jue Liu Tang [Pinyin: jué liú tāng, 決流湯, Break Water Decoction]:

黑醜	hēi chǒu	Seed of Pharbitis nil	2 qian
甘草	gān cǎo	Root of Glycyrrhiza uralensis	2 qian
肉桂	ròu guì	Bark of Cinnamonum cassia	3 fen
車前	chē qián	Seed of Plantago asiatica	1 liang

One dose gives an effluent of over one *dou* in volume, two doses cure the disease. Never administer the third dose, which is lethal. **Hēi chǒu** and **gān suí** are best in inducing diuresis, and **ròu guì** and **chē qián zǐ** lead fire to the bladder, which induces water without leaking qi4 and softens the strength of **hēi chǒu** and **gān suí**. After two doses, *Wu Ling San* [Pinyin: wǔ líng sǎn, 五苓散, Five Ling Powder] shall be used to recuperate the doses and finally *Liu Jun Zi Tang* [Pinyin: liù jūn zǐ tāng, 六君子湯, Six Gentle Medicinals Decoction] is applied to tonify the spleen. Salt should be strictly prohibited, otherwise death befalls.

The mimic use of *Wu Pi Yin* [Pinyin: wǔ pí yǐn, 五皮飲, Five Pi Decoction] by those mountebanks is totally useless.

氣臌

此證氣虛作腫，似水而實非水也，但按之不如泥耳。必先從腳面上腫起，後漸腫至身上，於是頭面皆腫者有之。此即謂之氣臌，宜於健脾行氣之中加引水之品。若以治水臌治之，是速之死也。方用：

白朮、茯苓、薏仁各壹兩，甘草、肉桂各壹分，枳殼伍分、人參、神麴、車前子、蘿蔔子各壹錢，山藥伍錢，水煎服。

初服若覺有礙，久之自有大功，三十劑而愈矣，亦忌食鹽、秋石。

Qi4-deficiency Tympanites

This disease has symptoms of qi4-deficiency edema as if caused by fluid accumulation though actually not. The body, which is not sludge-like if pressed, swells from the insteps and gradually reaches upward to patient's face and head sometimes. This is the so-called Qi4-deficiency Tympanites. It is proper to administer medicinals for spleen tonification and qi4 movement together with some for water conduction. If treated as ascites, the patient dies soon. Formula:

白朮	bái zhú	Rhizome of Atractylodes macrocephala	1 liang
茯苓	fú líng	Dried fungus of Poria cocos	1 liang
薏仁	yì rén	Seed kernel of Coix lachryma-jobi	1 liang
甘草	gān cǎo	Root of Glycyrrhiza uralensis	1 fen
肉桂	ròu guì	Bark of Cinnamonum cassia	1 fen
枳殼	zhǐ ké	Dried peel of Aurantii fructus	5 fen
人參	rén shēn	Root of Panax ginseng	1 qian
神麴	shén qū	Medicated leaven	1 qian
車前子	chē qián zǐ	Seed of Plantago asiatica	1 qian
蘿蔔子	luó bo zǐ	Raddish seed	1 qian
山藥	shān yào	Root of Dioscorea opposita	5 qian

Patients may doubt at the beginning sphere of medicine intake, but effectiveness of the decoction will be felt if time is given. Thirty doses cure, but salt and *prepared salt*[87] should be strictly prohibited.

---

[87] *prepared salt*: 秋石, "sal praeparatus", is prepared with gypsum and boy's urine.

蟲臌

此證小腹痛，四肢浮腫而未甚，面色紅而有白點，如蟲食之狀，是之謂蟲臌。方用消蟲神奇丹：

當歸、鱉甲、地栗粉各壹兩，雷丸、神麴、茯苓、白礬各叁錢，車前子伍錢　，水煎服。

一劑下蟲無數，二劑蟲盡臌消，不必三劑。但病好必用六君子湯去甘草調理。

Tympanites due to Parasitic Infestation

It has symptoms of pain in the lower abdomen, edema of the extremities though not the utmost type, red complexion with white spots in the shape of something eaten by worms. The prescription is *Xiao Chong Shen Qi Dan* [Pinyin: xiāo chóng shén qí dān, 消蟲神奇丹, Magic Worm-killing Pills]:

當歸	dāng guī	Root of Angelica polimorpha	1 liang
鳖甲	biē jiǎ	Dorsal shell of Amyda sinensis	1 liang
地栗粉	dì lì fěn	Powder of Waternut corm	1 liang
雷丸	léi wán	Dried Omphalia	3 qian
神麴	shén qū	Medicated leaven	3 qian

茯苓	fú líng	Dried fungus of Poria cocos	3 qian
白礬	bái fán	Alumen	3 qian
車前子	chē qián zǐ	Seed of Plantago asiatica	5 qian

The first dose kills countless worms, the second dispels tympanites, and the third dose is unnecessary. *Liu Jun Zi Tang* [Pinyin: liù jūn zǐ tāng, 六君子湯, Six Gentle Medicinals Decoction] (without **gān cǎo** in the formula) shall be prescribed for recuperation and complete recovery of patients.

血臌

此證或因跌閃而瘀血不散，或憂鬱而結血不行，或風邪而蓄血不散，留在腹中，致成血臌，飲食入胃不變精血，反去助邪，久則脹，脹成臌矣。倘以治水法逐之，而證非水，徒傷元氣；以治氣法治之，而又非氣，徒增飽滿。方用逐瘀湯：

水蛭（此物最難死，火燒經年，入水猶生，必須炒黃為末方妥）雷丸、紅花、枳殼、白芍、牛膝各叁錢，當歸貳兩，桃仁肆拾粒，水煎服。

一劑血盡而愈，切勿與二劑，當改四物湯調理，於補血内加白朮、茯苓、人參，補元氣而利水，自然全愈，否則恐成乾血之症。辨血臌惟腹脹如臌，而四肢手足並無臌意也。

Blood Tympanites

The symptom is caused by accumulated *static blood*[88] due to patient's fall or sprain, or blood stasis due to depression, or blood retention due to pathogens, all of which may stay in the abdomen to induce blood tympanites. Diets, instead of turning into essence and blood, assist pathogens, which induces distension that in turn turns into tympanites. It may harm the patient's source qi4 if treated as ascites and increases distension and fullness if treated as qi4-deficiency tympanites. The formula is *Zhu Yu Tang* [Pinyin: zhú yū tāng, 逐瘀湯, Decoction for *Breaking Blood and Expelling Stasis*[89]]:

水蛭 shuĭ zhì Dried body of Whitmania pigra 3 qian

[88] *static blood*: a pathological product of blood stagnation, including extravasated blood and the blood circulating sluggishly or blood congested in a viscus, all of which may turn into pathogenic factor, the same as blood stasis or stagnant blood.

[89] *break blood and expel stasis:* a therapeutic method to treat severe cases of blood stasis with intact health qi by using drastic blood activating medicinals.

(extremely tenacious, may resurrect back in water even after burning, it is a must to completely fry and grind it to powder)

雷丸	léi wán	Dried Omphalia	3 qian
紅花	hóng huā	Safflower	3 qian
枳殼	zhǐ ké	Dried peel of Aurantii fructus	3 qian
白芍	bái sháo	Root of Paeonia lactiflora	3 qian
牛膝	niú xī	Root of Achyranthes bidentata	3 qian
當歸	dāng guī	Root of Angelica polimorpha	2 liang
桃仁	táo rén	Seed of Prunus persica	40 pcs.

One does stops bleeding and cures; no more dose should be administered, but to change to *Si Wu Tang* [Pinyin: sì wù tāng,四物湯，Four-medicinal Decoction] for recuperation. Complete recovery is acquired if **bái zhú**, **fú líng**, and **rén shēn** are added for tonifying source qi4 and diverting water besides blood tonification. Otherwise, dryness and withering disease may form, which differs from blood tympanites with a symptom that only the abdomen of patient swells like a drum but not his extremities.

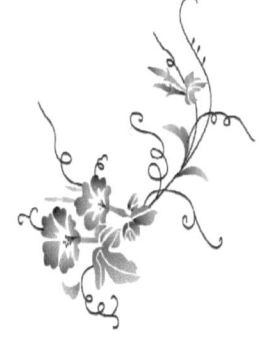

水證門

Chapter 10 Water Syndrome

水腫

此症土不能剋水也，方用：

牽牛、甘遂各叁錢，水煎服。

此症治法雖多，獨此方奇妙，其次雞屎醴亦效，雞屎醴治血臌尤效。

Edema

Edema[90] is attributed to the inability of earth in water control. Formula:

牽牛	qiān niú	Seed of Pharbitis nil	3 qian
甘遂	gān suí	Root of Gansui	3 qian

A lot of formulae aim at edema treatment, but this one has its own magic. Moreover, *Ji Shi Li* [Pinyin: jī shǐ lǐ, 雞屎醴, Prepared Wine of Chicken Feces] is also effective,

90 *edema*: any disease characterized by subcutaneous fluid retention.

though it is more applicable in treating tympanites due to blood stasis.

呃逆

此症乃水氣淩心包也，心包為水氣所淩，呃逆不止，號召五臟之氣，救水氣之犯心也，治法當利溼分水，方用：

茯神、薏仁各壹兩、蒼朮、白朮、人參各叁錢、芡實、丁香各伍錢、法製半夏陳皮各壹錢、吳萸三分，水煎服，二劑愈。

Hiccup

Hiccup[91] is due to water vapor's encroachment upon patient's heart. Once heart is encroached by water vapor, hiccup cannot stop and human body summons qi4 of the five viscera for help with resisting encroachment. Proper treatment is to drain dampness and divert water. Formula:

茯神	fú shén	Sclerotium of Poria cocos	1 liang
薏仁	yì rén	Seed kernel of Coix lachryma-jobi	1 liang
蒼朮	cāng zhú	Rhizome of Swordlike Atractylodes	3 qian

[91] *hiccup*: upward reversion of stomach qi with an involuntary movement of the diaphragm, causing a characteristic sound.

白朮 bái zhú Rhizome of Atractylodes macrocephala 3 qian

人參 rén shēn Root of Panax ginseng 3 qian

芡實 qiàn shí□ Seed of Euryale ferox 5 qian

丁香 dīng xiāng Flower bud of Syzygium aromaticum 5 qian

法製半夏 fǎ zhì bàn xià Prepared rhizome of Pinellia ternata 1 qian

陳皮 chén pí Peel of Citrus reticulata 1 qian

吳萸 wú yú Leaf of Trichotomous Evodia 3 fen

Two doses cure.

水結膀胱

此症目突口張，足腫氣喘，人以為不治之症，不知膀胱與腎，相為表裏，膀胱之開合，腎司其權，特通其腎氣而膀胱自通矣，方用通腎消水湯：

熟地、山藥、薏仁各壹兩、山萸壹錢伍分、茯神伍錢、肉桂、牛膝各壹錢、車前子叁錢，水煎服。

Bladder Water Congestion

This syndrome manifests itself with bulging eyes, open mouth, swollen feet and panting, which are often mistaken for the incurable diseases. People do not know that bladder and kidney have an interior-exterior relationship, and the kidney is in charge of the open-close movement of bladder. Therefore, if kidney qi4 is regulated, the bladder will function properly. The formula is *Tong Shen Xiao Shui Tang* [pinyin: tōng shèn xiāo shuǐ tāng, 通腎消水湯, Decoction for the Regulation of Kidney and Dispersion of Water]:

熟地	shú dì	Prepared root of Rehmannia glutinosa	1 liang
山藥	shān yào	Root of Dioscorea opposite	1 liang
薏仁	yì rén	Seed kernel of Coix lachryma-jobi	1 liang
山萸	shān yú	Fruit of Cornus officinalis	1 qian 5 fen
茯神	fú shén	Sclerotium of Poria cocos	5 qian
肉桂	ròu guì	Bark of Cinnamonum cassia	1 qian
牛膝	niú xī	Root of Achyranthes bidentata	1 qian
車前子	chē qián zǐ	Seed of Plantago asiatica	3 qian

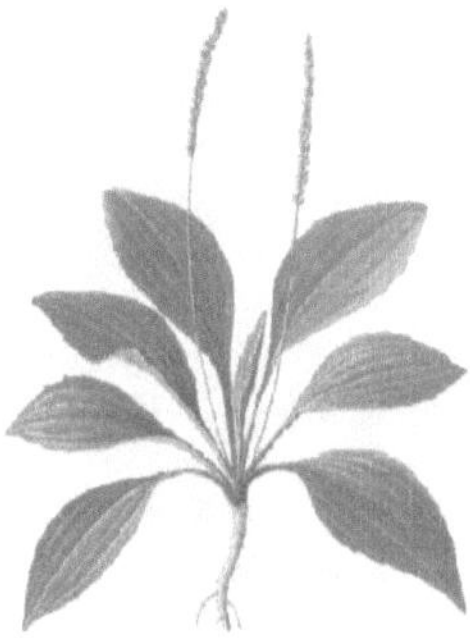

濕症

Chapter 11　Dampness Syndrome

黃症

此症外感之濕易治，內傷之濕難療，外感者利水則愈，若內傷之濕瀉水則氣消，發汗則精泄，必健脾行氣而後可也。方用：

白術、薏仁(各壹兩)、茵陳、黑梔(各三錢)、陳皮(伍分)，水煎服。

此方治內感之濕，不治外感之濕，若欲多服，去梔子。

Yellow Syndrome

As to *yellow syndrome*[92], dampness due to external contraction is easily treated through applying diuretics, while dampness due to internal detriment is hard to remedy since qi4 will be dispersed with purgation of water and the essence will be lost if diaphoresis is applied. Therefore, it is a must to fortify spleen and *move qi4*[93] beforehand. Formula:

---

[92] *yellow syndrome*: yellow syndrome might as well be understood as jaundice.

[93] *move qi4*: a therapeutic method of relieving stagnation of qi.

白術	bái zhú	Rhizome of Atractylodes macrocephala	1 liang
茯苓	fú líng	Dried fungus of Poria cocos	1 liang
薏仁	yì rén	Seed kernel of Coix lachryma-jobi	1 liang
茵陳	yīn chén	Seedling of Capillary Wormwood	3 qian
黑梔	hēi zhì	Fruit or root of Gardenia stenphylla Merr.	3 qian
陳皮	chén pí	Peel of Citrus reticulata	5 fen

This formula aims at treating dampness due to internal damage rather than the dampness of external contraction. For repeated dosages, **zhī zǐ** shall be left out.

瘅症

此證雖因風寒濕而來，亦因元氣之虛，邪治得趁虛而入，倘攻邪而不補正，則難愈矣。今於補正之中，佐以去風寒濕之品，而瘅如失矣。方用：

白術伍錢，人三三錢，茯苓壹兩，柴胡、附子、半夏各壹錢，陳皮伍分，水煎服。（經雲風寒濕三者合而成痹，此條原本瘅字，當是痹字之誤）

Heat Syndrome

This syndrome is attributed to invasions of wind, cold and dampness, though that the pathogens have taken advantage of qi4 deficiency is also ascribable. If the pathogens are attacked without tonifying healthy qi4, recovery is hard. In this formula, tonifying medicinals are assisted by those for dispelling cold and dampness, so the impediment is gone. Formula:

白術	bái zhú	Rhizome of Atractylodes macrocephala	5 qian
人三	rén sān	Root of Panax ginseng	3 qian
茯苓	fú líng	Dried fungus of Poria cocos	1 liang
柴胡	chái hú	Root of Bupleurum chinense	1 qian
附子	fù zǐ	Lateral root of Aconitum carmichaeli	1 qian
半夏	bàn xià	Rhizome of Pinellia ternata	1 qian
陳皮	chén pí	Peel of Citrus reticulata	5 fen

(Impediment is caused by combination of wind, cold and dampness, the title, therefore, should have been

Impediment Syndrome[94] instead of *Heat Syndrome*[95], which must be a wrong wording.)

傷濕

此證惡濕，身重足腫，小便短赤。方用：

澤瀉、豬苓各三錢，肉桂伍分，茯苓、白術各伍錢，柴胡、半夏、車前子各壹錢，水煎服，一劑愈。

Dampness Damage

Dampness damage[96] manifests itself with aversion to dampness, somatic heaviness, swollen feet and scanty dark urine. Formula:

澤瀉	zé xiè	Rhizome of Alisma plantago-aquatica	3 qian
豬苓	zhū líng	Agaric	3 qian

---

[94] *impediment disease*: a group of diseases caused by the invasion of wind, cold, dampness or heat pathogen on the meridian/channel involving muscles, sinews, bones and joints, manifested by local pain, soreness, heaviness, or hotness, and even articular swelling, stiffness and deformities, also referring to arthralgia.

[95] *impediment vs. heat*: the two characters 痹 and 癉 are similar in appearance, and might have been confused here.

[96] *Dampness damage*: a disease due to external contraction of dampness or obstruction of the stomach and intestines by dampness-turbidity.

肉桂	ròu guì	Bark of Cinnamonum cassia	5 fen
茯苓	fú líng	Dried fungus of Poria cocos	5 qian
白術	bái zhú	Rhizome of Atractylodes macrocephala	5 qian
柴胡	chái hú	Root of Bupleurum chinense	1 qian
半夏	bàn xià	Rhizome of Pinellia ternata	1 qian
車前子	chē qián zǐ	Seed of Plantago asiatica	1 qian

One dose of water decoction cures.

腳氣

今人以五苓散去濕，亦是正理，然不升其氣，而濕未必盡去也，必須提氣而水乃散也。方用：

黃耆壹兩，人三、白術各三錢，防風、肉桂、柴胡各壹錢，薏仁、芡實、白芍各伍錢，半夏貳錢，陳皮伍分，水煎服。

此方去濕之聖藥，防風用於黃耆之中，已足提氣而去濕，又助之柴胡舒氣，則氣自升騰。氣升則水散，白術、茯苓、薏仁、芡實俱是去濕之品，有不神效者乎？

Beriberi

It's a rightful treatment to use *Wuling San*[97] to dispell dampness nowadays. Nevertheless, if *middle qi4 is not upraised*[98], dampness will not be completely dispelled, and the middle qi4 must be upraised before water is dissipated. Formula:

黃耆	huáng qí	Root of Astragalus membranaceus	1 liang
人三	rén sān	Root of Panax ginseng□	3 qian
白術	bái zhú	Rhizome of Atractylodes macrocephala	3 qian
防風	fáng fēng	Root of Ledebouriella divaricata	1 qian
肉桂	ròu guì	Bark of Cinnamonum cassia	1 qian
柴胡	chái hú	Root of Bupleurum chinense	1 qian
薏仁	yì rén	Seed kernel of Coix lachryma-jobi	5 qian
芡實	qiàn shí□	Seed of Gordon Euryale	5 qian
白芍	bái sháo	Root of Paeonia lactiflora	5 qian
半夏	bàn xià	Rhizome of Pinellia ternata	2 qian
陳皮	chén pí	Peel of Citrus reticulata	5 fen

[97] Wuling San: Powder of five ingredients with poria.

[98] *upraise the middle q4i*: a therapeutic method to treat sunken middle qi4 by using qi-tonifying medicinals with upraising actions.

This is a sovereign remedy for dispelling dampness. Merely the usage of **huáng qí** with accompany of **fáng fēng** is competent in upraising middle qi4 to dispell dampness. **Chái hú** is as well added for its assistance in qi4 relaxation. Middle qi4 upraises therefore in its own right and as a result, the water dissipates. **Bái zhú**, **fú líng**, **yì rén** and **qiàn shí** are all known for their effectiveness in dispelling dampness, hence the formula's magic power.

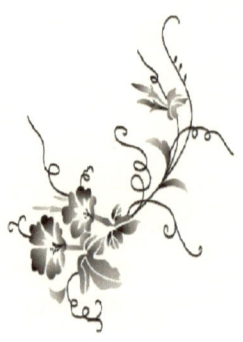

Fu Qing-zhu's Formula Book on Men's Diseases

Fù Qīng Zhǔ Nán Kē

傅青主男科

Book II

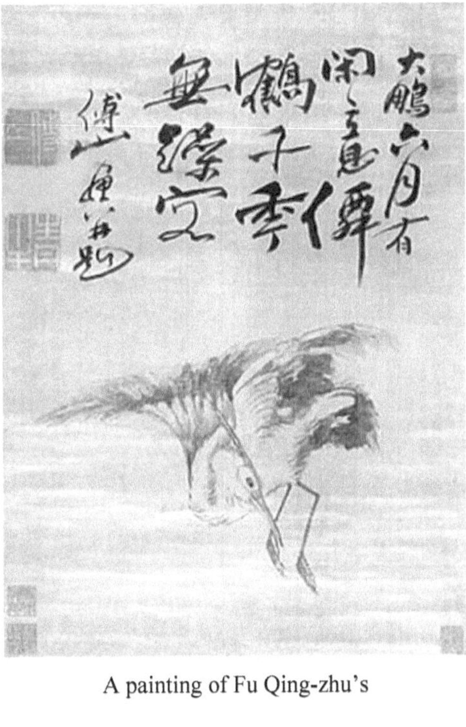

A painting of Fu Qing-zhu's

泄瀉門

Chapter 1　Diarrhea

瀉甚

一日五、六十回，傾腸而出，完穀不化，糞門腫痛，如火之熱，苟無以救之，必致立亡。方用截瀉湯：

薏仁、白芍各貳錢，山藥、車前子各壹兩，黃連、茯苓各伍錢，澤瀉、甘草各貳錢，肉桂參分、人參叁錢，水煎服。

Uttermost Diarrhea

Diarrhea occurs fifty or sixty times a day with symptoms of complete vacancy of the intestines, loose stool that contains indigested grains and swelling anus that hurts like burning. If proper treatment is not given, death befalls instantly. The prescription is *Jiexie Tang* [pinyin: jié xiè tāng, 截瀉湯, Decoction for Stopping Diarrhea]:

薏仁	yì rén	Seed kernel of Coix lachryma-jobi	2 qian
白芍	bái sháo	Root of Paeonia lactiflora	2 qian

山藥 shān yào Root of Dioscorea opposita 1 liang

車前子 chē qián zǐ Seed of Plantago asiatica 1 liang

黃連 huáng lián Rhizome of Coptis chinensis 5 qian

茯苓 fú líng Dried fungus of Poria cocos 5 qian

澤瀉 zé xiè Rhizome of Alisma plantago-aquatica 2 qian

甘草 gān cǎo Root of Glycyrrhiza uralensis 2 qian

肉桂 ròu guì Bark of Cinnamonum cassia 3 fen

人參 rén shén Root of Panax ginseng 3 qian

水瀉

方用：白朮壹兩，車前子伍錢，水煎服。此方補腎健脾，利水去溼，治瀉神效。

泄瀉之證，皆由于膀胱不能化氣，胃中所納水穀不得分消，直由大腸而出。故以利小便為主，與傷寒下利自利，大相懸殊，須察之。

Watery Diarrhea

Formula:

白术 bái zhú Rhizome of Atractylodes macrocephala 1 liang

車前子 chē qián zǐ Seed of Plantago asiatica 5 qian

This formula tonifies kidney and fortifies spleen. It promotes diuresis and dispels dampness, and is miraculously effective to diarrhea treatment.

Diarrhea is all attributed to bladder's failure to transform qi4 and the water and food intake is not properly digested in stomach but goes directly out of the large intestine. This formula, therefore, focuses on promoting urination, which is diametrically different from those treating *clear-food diarrhea*[99] and *spontaneous diarrhea*[100] of cold damage. This point should be carefully observed.

火瀉

完穀不化，飲食下喉即出，日夜數十次，甚至百次，人皆知為熱也，然而熱之生也何故？生於腎中之水衰不能制火，使胃土關門，不守於上下，所以直進而直出也。論其勢之急迫，似乎宜治其標，然治其標而不能使火之驟降，必須急補腎中之水，使火有可居之地，而後不致上騰也。方用：

熟地、白芍各參兩，山萸、茯苓、甘草、車前子各壹

99 *clear-food diarrhea*: frequent discharge of fluid stools containing undigested food, the same as undigested food diarrhea.

100 *spontaneous diarrhea:* diarrhea not attributable to purgation.

兩，肉桂參分，水煎服。

此方補腎之藥，非止瀉之品，然而止瀉之妙，捷如桴鼓矣，世人安知此也。

Fire Diarrhea

Fire diarrhea has symptoms of loose stool that contains indigested grain, almost instant defecation upon food intake for tens or even a hundred times a day. Normally it is thought of as heat syndrome, but where does the heat come from? It originates in a situation that kidney water cannot restrain fire, which closes the door to stomach earth, and healthy qi4 is not retained in the upper or lower body so that food intake goes directly out. As far as the situation is concerned, it seems appropriate to treat the tip, which, however, cannot downbear fire rapidly. Therefore, kidney water should be urgently tonified in order that the fire inhabits in its own abode and will not flame upward. Formula:

熟地	shú dì	Prepared root of Rehmannia glutinosa	3 liang
白芍	bái sháo	Root of Paeonia lactiflora	3 liang
山萸	shān yú	Fruit of Cornus officinalis	1 liang

茯苓	fú líng	Dried fungus of Poria cocos	1 liang
甘草	gān cǎo	Root of Glycyrrhiza uralensis	1 liang
車前子	chē qián zǐ	Seed of Plantago asiatica	1 liang
肉桂	ròu guì	Bark of Cinnamonum cassia	3 fen

This is a kidney-tonifying formula instead of a diarrhea-checking one. It checks diarrhea as quickly as the drumbeats for reporting victory of war battles, which is quite beyond the knowledge of some common practioners.

水瀉

此乃純是下清水，非言下痢也。痢無止法，豈瀉水亦無止法乎？故人患水瀉者，急宜止遏。方用：

白朮伍錢，茯苓叁錢，吳萸五分，車前子、五味子各壹錢，水煎服。

Watery Diarrhea

This is a diarrhea of exclusively clear water rather than dysentery. Dysentery cannot be stopped, but watery diarrhea is quite another case. It can be checked rapidly. Formula:

白术	bái zhú	Rhizome of Atractylodes macrocephala	5 qian
茯苓	fú líng	Dried fungus of Poria cocos	3 qian
吳萸	wú yú	Foliage of Trichotomous Evodia	5 fen
車前子	chē qián zǐ	Seed of Plantago asiatica	1 qian
五味子	wǔ wèi zǐ	Fruit of Schisandra chinensis	1 qian

泄瀉吞酸

泄瀉，寒也，吞酸，火也，似乎寒熱殊而治法異矣。不知吞酸雖熱，由於肝氣之鬱結，泄瀉雖寒，由於肝木之剋脾，苟用一方以治水鬱，又一方以培脾土，土必大崩，木必大彫矣，不若一方而兩治之為愈也，方用：

白芍伍錢、柴胡、車前子各壹錢、茯苓叁錢、神麴、陳皮、甘草各伍分，水煎服。

此方妙在白芍以舒肝木之鬱，木鬱一舒，上不剋胃，下不剋脾，又有茯苓車前，以分消水溼之氣，則水盡從小便出，而何有餘水以吞酸，剌汁以泄瀉哉。

Diarrhea with Acid Regurgitation

Diarrhea is of cold pathogen, while *acid regurgitation*[101] is of fire. It seems that the therapies should

[101] *acid regurgitation*: swallowing of acid contents regurgitated from the

vary since cold is different from heat. People do not know that acid regurgitation as a heat disease is due to liver qi4 depression; Diarrhea, as a cold one, is due to liver wood's restraint of spleen. If one formula is employed to treat water depression and another is used to cultivate spleen earth, the earth will collapse and the wood will totally wither as a result. Treatment is attained only by a formula capable of tackling both symptoms. Formula:

白芍	bái sháo	Root of Paeonia lactiflora	5 qian
柴胡	chái hú	Root of Bupleurum chinense	1 qian
車前子	chē qián zǐ	Seed of Plantago asiatica	1 qian
茯苓	fú líng	Dried fungus of Poria cocos	3 qian
神麴	shén qū	Medicated leaven	5 fen
陳皮	chén pí	Peel of Citrus reticulata	5 fen
甘草	gān cǎo	Root of Glycyrrhiza uralensis	5 fen

The beauty of this formula consists in its employment of **bái sháo** for soothing depressed liver wood. If liver wood is soothed, it restrains neither the upper stomach nor the lower spleen.

stomach to the throat.

Moreover, **fú ling** and **chē qián zǐ** are used to separately eliminate dampness qi4 and the water is drained as urine. As a result, there is no more water for acid regurgitation, nor is there any for the rushing stool of diarrhea.

痢疾門

Chapter 2 Dysentery

火邪內傷辨

火邪之血，色必鮮紅，脈必洪緩，口必渴而飲冷水，小便必澀而赤濁。內傷之血色不鮮而紫暗，或微紅淡白，脈必細而遲，或浮濇而空，口不渴，即渴而喜飲熱湯，小便不赤不澀，即赤而不熱不濁。此訣也。

痢疾以調達氣血為主，痢門以芍藥湯為總方，芍藥湯偏於涼，用之每不得效。此諸方雖歸芍木香，卻分證而用芩、連，不用大黃，可云盡善盡美。

Differentiation between Pathogenic Fire and Internal Damage

Bleeding caused by pathogenic fire is always scarlet red in color. The sufferer, whose pulse is invariably surging and relaxed, always has symptoms of thirst for cold water, difficult urination and turbid urine reddish in color. Bleeding of internal damage, on the other hand, is not bright but dull purple or reddish white in color. The patient, whose pulse is always fine and slow, or floating, rough and hollow, is not thirsty. Even if he is, he is for hot water. His urination is neither reddish in color nor difficult. Even if the urine is reddish, it is not hot or turbid. This is the crux.

Treatment of dysentery relies chiefly on blood and qi4 adjustment, the principle formula for dysenteric diseases is *Shaoyao Tang* [pinyin: sháo yào tāng, 芍藥湯, Peony Decoction] which tends to be cool in property and often fails to gain satisfactory results. Though belonging to formulae using **sháo yào** and **mù xiāng**, we should differentiate the syndromes and adopt **huáng qín** and **huáng lián** instead of **dà huáng**, so as to reach perfection.

痢疾

此證感溼熱而成，紅白相見，如膿如血，至危至急者也。茍用涼藥止血，熱藥攻邪，俱非善治之法。方用：

白芍、當歸各貳兩，枳殼、檳榔各貳錢，滑石叁錢，廣木香、來服子、甘草各壹錢，水煎服。一二劑收功。

此方妙在用歸、芍至二兩之多，則肝血有餘，不去剋脾土，自然大腸有傳送之功，加之枳殼、檳榔，俱逐穢去積之品，尤能於補中用攻，而滑石、甘草、木香，調達於遲速之間，不疾不徐，使瘀滯盡下也。其餘些小痢疾，減半用之，無不奏功。此方不論紅、白痢疾，痛與不痛，服之皆神效。又方：

當歸壹兩，黃芩柒分酒洗，蒼朮、厚樸、大復皮、陳皮各壹錢，水二碗，煎一碗，頓服。

Dysentery

Dysentery, which is the result of damp heat contraction, has a perilous symptom of reddish white colored dysenteric *stool of blood and pus*[102]. Neither bleeding-stopping medicinals cool in property nor pathogen-attacking ones hot in property is the proper treatment. Formula:

白芍	bái sháo	Root of Paeonia lactiflora	2 liang
當歸	dāng guī	Root of Angelica polimorpha	2 liang
枳殼	zhǐ ké	Dried peel of Aurantii fructus	2 qian
檳榔	bīng láng	Fruit of Areca catechu	2 qian
滑石	huá shí	Talcum	3 qian
廣木香	guǎng mù xiāng	Root of Aucklandia lappa	1qian
來服子	lái fú zǐ	RadishSeed	1 qian

102 *stool of pus and blood:* passage of blood, pus and mucus together with stool, a symptom usually indicating dysentery.

甘草 gān cǎo Root of Glycyrrhiza uralensis 1 qian

One or two doses will cure.

The beauty of this formula consists in its employment of heavy doses of **bái sháo** and **dāng guī**, which makes it possible that liver blood is in surplus and not to restrain spleen earth, and the large intestine in turn conveys successfully. Moreover, **zhǐ ké** and **bīng láng**, two medicinals for dispelling filth and removing accumulation, are well applied in the middle qi4 tonification; **Huá shí**, **gān cǎo** and **mù xiāng** are used to attack pathogens, regulate the lateness or earliness of the efficacy to make it neither expeditious nor dilatory, and all stasis and stagnation are purged. Other minor dysenteric diseases are all cured with half dosage. Dysentery of whether white or red, painful or painless, is cured upon intake of the decoction without exception. Another formula:

當歸 dāng guī Root of Angelica polimorpha 1 liang
黃芩 huáng qín Root of Scutellaria baicalensis (wine-washed) 7 fen

蒼朮 cāng zhú Rhizome of Swordlike Atractylodes 1 qian

厚樸 hòu pò Bark of Magnolia officinalis 1 qian

大復皮 dà fù pí Dried peel of Pericarpium Arecae 1qian

陳皮 chén pí Peel of Citrus reticulata 1 qian

Two bowls of water is decocted into one bowl of decoction for taking at one draft.

血痢

凡血痢腹痛者，火也。方用：

歸尾、白芍各壹兩，黃連叁錢，枳殼、木香、來服子各貳錢，水煎服。

Blood Dysentery

Blood dysentery with the symptom of painful abdomen is due to fire pathogen. Formula:

歸尾 guī wěi Prepared root of Radix Angelicae Sinensis 1 liang

白芍 bái sháo Root of Paeonia lactiflora 1 liang

黃連 huáng lián Rhizome of Coptis chinensis 3 qian

枳殼 zhǐ ké Dried peel of Aurantii fructus 2 qian

木香 mù xiāng Root of Aucklandia lappa 2 qian

來服子	lái fú zǐ	Radish Seed	2 qian

寒痢

凡痢腹不痛者，寒也。方用：

白芍、當歸各叁錢，枳殼、檳榔、甘草、來服子各壹錢，水煎服。

前方治壯實之人，火邪挾溼者；此方治寒痢，腹不痛者。更有內傷勞倦，與中氣虛寒之人脾不攝血而成血痢者，當用理中湯加木香肉桂；或用補中益氣湯加熟地、炒乾薑治之而始愈也。

Cold Dysentery

Dysentery without abdominal pain is due to cold pathogen. Formula:

白芍	bái sháo	Root of Paeonia lactiflora	3 q i a n
當歸	dāng guī	Root of Angelica polimorpha	3 qian
枳殼	zhǐ ké	Dried peel of Aurantii fructus	1 qian
檳榔	bīng láng	Fruit of Areca catechu	1 qian
甘草	gān cǎo	Root of Glycyrrhiza uralensis	1 qian

來服子 lái fú zǐ Radish Seed 1 qian

The aforesaid formula treats strong and healthy patient with fire pathogen complicated by dampness, while this one treats cold dysentery patient without abdominal pain. Moreover, for those of internal damage, fatigue and middle qi4 *deficiency cold*[103], and those whose spleen fails to control blood that causes blood dysentery, either *Lizhong Tang* [pinyin: lǐ zhōng tāng, 理中湯, Decoction for Mid Energizer Regulation] added with **mù xiāng** and **ròu guì**, or *Buzhong Yiqi Tang* [pinyin: bǔ zhōng yì qì tāng, 補中益氣湯, Central Qi4 Tonification Decoction] added with **shú dì** and **chǎo gān jiāng** [Sand-fried Common ginger] is recommended. These two formulae initiate the cure of cold dysentery.

---

103 *deficiency cold*: a pathological change arising when yang qi4 becomes insufficient and fails to provide adequate warmth.

大小便門

Chapter 3 Urination and Defecation

大便不通

此症人以為大腸燥也，誰知是肺氣燥乎，蓋肺燥則清肅之氣，不能下行於大腸，而腎經之水，僅足自顧，又何能旁流以潤潤哉，方用：

熟地、元參各參兩、升麻三錢、火麻仁壹錢、牛乳壹碗，水二碗，煎六分，將牛乳同調服之，一二劑必大便矣。

此方不在潤大腸而在補腎及清肺，夫大腸居於下流，最難獨治，必須從腎以潤之，從肺以清之，啟其上竅，則下竅自然流動通利矣，此下病上治之法也。

Constipation

Normally regarded as the result of dryness in large intestine, constipation is in fact a symptom of dryness of lung qi4 in that clear and cleansing qi4 cannot go down into the large intestine in condition of lung dryness. Moreover, water of *kidney meridian*[104] merely suffices itself, how

---

[104] *kidney meridian*: One of the twelve regular meridians which begins on the plantar tip of the small toe and travels to yongquan (KI1) in the

come the nourishment and moistening of the offshoots? Formula:

熟地	shú dì	Prepared root of Rehmannia glutinosa	3 liang
元參	yuán shēn	Root of Scrophularia ningpoensis	3 liang
升麻	shēng má	Rhizome of Cimifuga foetida	3 qian
火麻仁	huǒ má rén	Seed of Cannabis sativa	1 qian
牛乳	niú rǔ	Milk of Bos taurus domesticus	1 bowlful

Two bowls of water is decocted into sixty percent of its original volume, and mix with milk for intake. Just one or two doses are enough to *relax the bowels*[105].

This formula focuses not on moistening the large intestine but on kidney tonification and lung clearance. Large intestine lies in the lower body, the hardest part to treat alone. Treatment therefore, must be sought from moistening kidney and clearing lung so as to open the upper orifices. In this way, the lower orifices naturally function to

---

center of the sole, continues along the medial side of the lower limb to the symphysis pubis, turns internally to the kidney and bladder, and back to the symphysis pubis, ascending along the abdomen and chest up to shufu (KI27) in the depression between the first rib and the lower border of the clavicle, with 27 acupuncture points on either side.

105 *relax the bowels*: therapeutic method for relieving constipation.

defecate. This is the method of treating lower diseases from the upper.

實症大便不通

方用：

大黃伍錢，歸尾壹兩，升麻伍分，蜂蜜半盃，水煎服。此方大黃泄利，當歸以潤之，仍以為君，雖泄而不至十分猛烈，不致有亡險之弊，況有升麻以提之，則泄中有留，又何必過慮哉？

此方之妙在升麻，味能化板為靈，啟其上竅則下竅自流，每以筆管汲硯池水比之，指按管則得水，指啟則水落硯上，淺而易明，嶽診小便不通，以青龍湯之薑、細、味主之，亦此意也。 此方比大承氣和平，然陽明燥糞，非大承氣不可，此方當歸重用，溫潤而不猛也，此方從八味地黃悟出。

Constipation of Excess

Formula:

大黃	dà huáng	Root of Rheum palmatum	5 qian
歸尾	guī wěi	Prepared root of Radix Angelicae Sinensis	1 liang
升麻	shēng má	Rhizome of Cimifuga foetida	5 fen

蜂蜜 fēng mì Honey of Polistes mandarinus half cupful

In this formula, **Dà huáng** is used to purge with the lubricant function of monarchic **dāng guī**, so that the purgation is not too severe to induce a risk of death. Let along the upraising function of **shēng má**, which retains in the process of purgation. There is no need for worry.

The wisdom of this formula lies in its use of **shēng má**, which breaks the deadlock by opening upper orifices and as a result the lower orifices open by themselves. An easily understandable and comparable fact is to draw water with a writing brush from the inkstone. Water is held in the bamboo pipe if a finger is pressed against the top of the pipe, and water drops down when the finger lifts. *Yue*'s[106] treatment of difficult urination with *Qinglong Tang* [pinyin: qīng long tāng, 青龍湯, Green Dragon Decoction], which chiefly employs **gān jiāng** and **xì xīn** has the same purpose. This formula is milder than *Da Chengqi* [pinyin: dà chéng qì, 大承氣, Major Drastic Purgative Decoction]. However, *Da Chengqi* must be applied for purging the dry filth of

---

106 *yue*: a abbreviation for the famous doctor Zhang Jingyue of Ming dynasty.

Yangming. The heavy dosage of **dāng guī** in this formula warmly moistens but without strong efficacy. The author deduced this formula from *Bawei Dihuang* [pinyin: bā wèi dì huáng, 八味地黃, Decoction of Eight Drugs including Rehmannia].

虛症大便不通

人有病後大便秘者。方用：

熟地、元參、當歸各壹兩，川芎伍錢，桃仁拾粒，紅花、大黃各三錢，火麻仁壹錢，蜂蜜半盃，水煎服。

Constipation of Deficiency

Some patients suffer from constipation during their convalescence. Formula:

熟地	shú dì	Prepared root of Rehmannia glutinosa	1 liang
元參	yuán shēn	Root of Scrophularia ningpoensis	1 liang
當歸	dāng guī	Root of Angelica polimorpha	1 liang
川芎	chuān xiōng	Root of Ligusticum wallichii	5 qian
桃仁	táo rén	Seed of Prunus persica	10 pieces
紅花	hóng huā	Safflower	3 qian

大黃	dà huáng	Root of Rheum palmatum	3 qian
火麻仁	huǒ má rén	Seed of Cannabis sativa	1 qian
蜂蜜	fēng mì	Honey of Polistes mandarinus	half cupful

小便不通

膀胱之氣化不行，即小便不通，似乎治膀胱也，然而治法全不在膀胱。方用：人參、茯苓、蓮子各三錢，白果貳錢，甘草、肉桂、車前子、王不留行各壹錢，水煎服。

此方妙在用人參、肉桂，蓋膀胱必得氣化而出，氣化者何？心包絡之氣也。既用參桂而氣化行矣，尤妙在用白果，人多不識此意，白果通任督之脈，走膀胱而引群藥；況車前子、王不留行，盡下洩之品，服之而前陰有不利者乎？

又方：

熟地壹兩，山藥、丹皮、澤瀉、肉桂、車前子各壹錢，山萸肆錢，水煎服。

此方不去通小便而專治腎水，腎中有水，而膀胱之氣，自然行矣。蓋膀胱之開合，腎司其權也。

Difficult Urination

Bladder's failure of *qi4 transformation*[107] results in difficult urination. It seems that bladder shall be treated, though it is not all about bladder. Formula:

人參	rén shén	Root of Panax ginseng	3 qian
茯苓	fú líng	Dried fungus of Poria cocos	3 qian
蓮子	lián zĭ	Lotus seed	3 qian
白果	bái guŏ	Seed of Semen Ginkgo	2 qian
甘草	gān căo	Root of Glycyrrhiza uralensis	1 qian
肉桂	ròu guì	Bark of Cinnamonum cassia	1 qian
車前子	chē qián zĭ	Seed of Plantago asiatica	1 qian
王不留行	wáng bù liú xíng	Seed of Semen Vaccariae	1 qian

The wisdom of this formula consists in its employment of **rén shén** and **ròu guì**. In order to micturate, the bladder must have qi4 transformation. What does it transform? It is qi4 of the pericardium. Besides the formula's employment of **rén shén** and **ròu guì** for qi4 transformation, **Bái guŏ** is

[107] *qi4 transformation*: a general term referring to various changes through the activity of qi4, namely the metabolism and mutual transformation between essence, qi4, blood and fluids.

marvelously used to unblock the *conception vessel*[108] and the *governor vessel*[109], which leads efficacy of the medicinals through the bladder. People rarely understand this point. Moreover, **chē qián zǐ** and **wáng bù liú xíng** are both medicinals for purgation, and may benefit the *anterior yin*[110] if used.

Another formula:

熟地 shú dì Prepared root of Rehmannia glutinosa 1 liang

---

[108] *conception vessel*: One of the eight extra meridians which originates in the lower abdomen, exists at huiyin (CV1), a point in the center of perineum, and ascends the midline of the abdominal wall and chest to chengjiang (CV24), midpoint of the mentolabial sulcus. The internal portion of this meridian/channel ascends from chengjiang (CV24), encircling the mouth and traveling to the eyes. Another branch travels internally from the pelvic cavity and ascends the spine to the throat, also called controlling vessel.

[109] *governor vessel*: One of the eight extra meridians which originates in the lower abdomen and exits at changqiang (GV1), a point at the back of the anus, sending 1 branch forward to huiyin (CV1). The main portion of the meridian/channel ascends along the midline of the back to the top of the head and then descends along the midline of the face down to yinjiao (GV28), a point between the upper lip and the upper gum in the labia frenum, also called governing vessel.

[110] *anterior yin:* external genitalia including the external orifice ofurethra.

山藥	shān yào	Root stock of Dioscorea opposita	1 qian
丹皮	dān pí	Bark of the root of Paeonia suffruticosa	1 qian
澤瀉	zé xiè	Rhizome of Alisma plantago-aquatica	1 qian
肉桂	ròu guì	Bark of Cinnamonum cassia	1 qian
車前子	chē qián zǐ	Seed of Plantago asiatica	1 qian
山萸	shān yú	Fruit of Cornus officinalis	4 qian

Instead of unblocking the urination, this formula dwells on the treatment of kidney water. With ample kidney water, qi4 of the bladder will naturally flow since kidney is in charge of the open and close of bladder.

大小便不通

方用：

頭髮燒灰研末，用三指一撚，入熱水半碗，飲之立通。

又方：

蜜一茶盃，皮硝一兩，黃酒一茶盃，大黃一錢，溫服神效。

Dual Blockage of Urination and Defecation

Formula:

Human hair is burned and ground to powder. One pinch

of the ash is mixed with half bowl of hot water for drinking. It unblocks immediately.

Another Formula:

Decoct one teacup of bee honey, one liang of **pí xiāo**, one cupful of rice wine, and one qian of **dà huáng**. Intake of the warm decoction brings about miraculous efficacy.

厥證門

Chapter 4 Syncope

寒厥

此症手足必青紫，飲水必吐，腹必痛，喜火熨之，方用：人參叁錢、白朮壹兩，附子、肉桂、吳萸各壹錢，水煎服。

Cold Syncope

Patient invariably has symptoms of bluish purple extremities, vomit at water drinking, painful abdomen that relieves if pressed against a hot object. Formula:

人參	rén shén	Root of Panax ginseng	3 qian
白朮	bái zhú	Rhizome of Atractylodes macrocephala	1 liang
附子	fù zǐ	Lateral root of Aconitum carmichaeli	1 qian
肉桂	ròu guì	Bark of Cinnamonum cassia	1 qian
吳萸	wú yú	Foliage of Trichotomous Evodia	1 qian

熱厥

此證手足雖寒而不青紫，飲水不吐，火熨之腹必痛，一時手足厥逆，痛不可忍。人以為四肢之風證也，誰知是心中熱蒸，外不能洩，故四肢手足則寒，而胸腹皮熱如火。方用：

柴胡叁錢，當歸、黃連、炒梔各貳錢，荊芥、半夏、枳殼各壹錢，水煎服，二劑愈。又方：

白芍壹兩，黑梔叁錢，陳皮、柴胡各壹錢，花粉貳錢，水煎服。以白芍為君，取入肝而平木也。

此證熱在於肝，前方之柴胡、當歸，後方之白芍皆肝藥也。

Heat Syncope

Patients with the syndrome have cold extremities though not bluish purple in color and patients do not vomit at water drinking. Abdominal pain is felt if pressed against a hot object. Patients may occasionally have reversal cold of extremities with intolerable pain. People may think it is a wind syndrome of extremities, but they are ignorant of the fact that the symptom is caused by the heat-steaming of the heart which cannot be purged externally. Patients have cold extremities and their skin of the chest and abdomen is as hot as fire. Formula:

柴胡	chái hú	Root of Bupleurum chinense	3 qian
當歸	dāng guī	Root of Angelica polimorpha	2 qian
黃連	huáng lián	Rhizome of Coptis chinensis	2 qian
炒梔	chǎo zhì	Stir-baked fruit of Gardenia jasminoides	2 qian
荊芥	jīng jiè	Foliage of Schizonepeta tenuifolia	1 qian
半夏	bàn xià	Rhizome of Pinellia ternata	1 qian
枳殼	zhǐ ké	Dried peel of Aurantii fructus	1 qian

In two doses the disease cures. Another formula:

白芍	bái sháo	Root of Paeonia lactiflora	1 liang
黑梔	hēi zhì	Fruit or root of Gardenia stenphylla Merr.	3 qian
陳皮	chén pí	Peel of Citrus reticulata	1 qian
柴胡	chái hú	Root of Bupleurum chinense	1qian
花粉	huā fěn	Seed of Trichosanthes kirilowii	2 qian

The formula employs **bái sháo** as monarch, efficacy of which enters the liver and pacifies the wood.

The syndrome has its heat on liver, and **chái hú** and **dāng guī** of the former formula as well as **bái sháo** of the latter are all medicinals for liver.

屍厥

此證一時猝倒，不省人事，乃氣虛而痰迷心也。補氣化痰而已。方用：

人參、半夏、南星各三錢，白朮伍錢，附子伍分，白芥子壹錢，水煎服。又方：

蒼朮三錢，水煎，灌之必吐，吐後則愈，蓋蒼朮陽藥，善能祛風，故有奇效。凡見鬼者用之更效。

Cadaverous Coma

Sufferers of this symptom fall down unconsciously all of sudden. This is due to qi4 deficiency and *phlegm clouding the pericardium*[111]. It is a proper treatment to tonfiy qi4 and resolve the phlegm. Formula:

人參	rén shén	Root of Panax ginseng	3 qian
半夏	bàn xià	Rhizome of Pinellia ternata	3qian
南星	nán xīng	Rhizome of Pinallia	3 qian

[111] *phlegm clouding the pericardium*: a pathological change in which phlegm causes mental confusion; the same as phlegm confounding the orifices of the heart.

白术 bái zhú Rhizome of Atractylodes macrocephala 5 qian

附子 fù zǐ Lateral root of Aconitum carmichaeli 5 fen

白芥子 bái jiè zǐ Seed of Brassica alba 1 qian

Another formula:

蒼朮 cāng zhú Rhizome of Swordlike Atractylodes 3 qian

Patient invariably vomits upon intake of the decoction, but recovers soon. The reason is that **cāng zhú**, a medicinal of yang tonifying property, is good at dispelling wind, hence its miraculous effect. This formula is more applicable to those who have seen ghosts.

厥症

人有忽然發厥，閉目撒手，喉中有聲，有一日死者，有二三日死者，此厥多犯神明，然亦素有痰氣而發也。治法宜攻其痰而開心竅。方用起迷丹：

人參、半夏各伍錢，菖蒲貳錢，兔絲子壹兩，茯苓、皂莢各叁錢，生薑壹錢，甘草叁分，水煎服。

Syncope

People who have a sudden attack of syncope close their eyes and let go of their hands, their throats grunt. Some die in a single day, while others die in two or three days. Though in most cases it is syncope of transgression against *bright spirit*[112], there might as well be cases of spasm of chronicle pathogenic phlegm. The proper prescription is to attack phlegm to open up pericardium. The formula is *Qimi Dan* [pinyin: qǐ mí dān, 起迷丹, Loss-relieving Pellet]:

人參	rén shén	Root of Panax ginseng	5 qian
半夏	bàn xià	Rhizome of Pinellia ternata	5 qian
菖蒲	chāng pú	Rhizome of Acorus gramineus	2 qian
兔絲子	tù sī zǐ	Seed of Cuscuta chinensis	1 liang
茯苓	fú líng	Dried fungus of Poria cocos	3 qian
皂莢	zào jiá	Fruit of Gleditsia sinensis	3 qian
生薑	shēng jiāng	Fresh root of Zingiber officinale	1 qian
甘草	gān cǎo	Root of Glycyrrhiza uralensis	3 fen

氣虛猝倒

人有猝然昏倒，迷而不悟，喉中有痰，人以為風也，誰知是氣虛乎，若作風治，無不死者，此症蓋因平日不慎

[112] *bright spirit*: all the human life activities including mind, will, mood and thinking, governed by the heart.

女色，精虧以致氣衰，又加不慎起居，而有似乎風者，其實非風也。 方用：

人參、黃耆、白朮各壹兩，茯苓伍錢、菖蒲、附子各壹錢、半夏貳錢、白芥子叁錢，水煎服。

此方補氣而不治風，消痰而不耗氣，一劑神定，二劑痰消，三劑全愈。

Cataplexy of Qi4 Deficiency

Patient may faint all of sudden. Being unconscious, the patient with phlegm in throat may die once treated as wind, though it is qi4 deficiency. The symptom can be traced up to qi4 debilitation of essence depletion, a result of imprudent sexual life. If combined with an irregular life of patient, it would appear as wind, though not in fact. Formula:

人參	rén shén	Root of Panax ginseng	1 liang
黃耆	huáng qí	Root of Astragalus membranaceus	1 liang
白朮	bái zhú	Rhizome of Atractylodes macrocephala	1 liang
茯苓	fú líng	Dried fungus of Poria cocos	5 qian
菖蒲	chāng pú	Rhizome of Acorus gramineus	1 qian
附子	fù zǐ	Lateral root of Aconitum carmichaeli	1 qian

半夏	bàn xià	Rhizome of Pinellia ternata	2 qian
白芥子	bái jiè zǐ	Seed of Brassica alba	3 qian

This formula tonifies qi4 instead of treating wind, and resolves phlegm without consuming qi4. The first dose settles the spirit of patient, and the second dose resolves the phlegm and the third cures.

陰虛猝倒

此證有腎中之水虛而不上交於心者，又有肝氣燥不能生心之火者，此皆陰虛而能令人猝倒者也。方用再甦丹：

熟地貳兩，山萸、元參、麥冬、五味子各壹兩，柴胡、菖蒲各壹錢，茯苓伍錢，白芥子叁錢，水煎服。

此方補腎水，滋肺氣、安心通竅、瀉火消痰、實有神功，十劑全愈。

此證切實為陰虛者，當此人身本瘦，面部以下青黑，倒時微喘，目不能瞑。

Cataplexy of Yin Deficiency

As for this syndrome, both the case that deficient kidney water cannot upraise to interact with the heart and the case thatdry liver qi4 cannot light heart fire, are regarded as yin deficiency cataplexy. The prescription is *Zaisu Dan* [pinyin: zài sū dān, 再甦丹, Consciousness Regaining Pellet]:

熟地	shú dì	Prepared root of Rehmannia glutinosa	2 liang
山萸	shān yú	Fruit of Cornus officinalis	1 liang
元參	yuán shēn	Root of Scrophularia ningpoensis	1 liang
麥冬	mài dōng	Tuber of Ophiopogon japonicus	1 liang
五味子	wǔ wèi zǐ	Fruit of Schisandra chinensis	1 liang
柴胡	chái hú	Root of Bupleurum chinense	1 qian
菖蒲	chāng pú	Rhizome of Acorus gramineus	1 qian
茯苓	fú líng	Dried fungus of Poria cocos	5 qian
白芥子	bái jiè zǐ	Seed of Brassica alba	3 qian

This formula aims at kidney water tonification and lung qi4 enrichment. It purges fire and resolves phlegm in a miraculous way. Ten doses cure. If patient's pulse is taken affirmatively to be a yin deficiency, he must be thin, and has a bluish dark color of his body under the neck, as well as insomnia with slight panting.

陽虛猝倒

人有心中火虛，不能下交於腎而猝倒者，陽虛也。方用：

人參、白朮、生棗仁各壹兩，茯神伍錢，附子、甘草各壹錢，生半夏叁錢，水煎服。藥下喉，則痰靜而氣出矣，連服數劑，則安然如故。此證又有胃熱不能安心之火而猝倒者，亦陽虛也。方用：

人參、元參各壹兩，石膏、花粉各伍錢，麥冬叁錢，菖蒲壹錢，水煎服。一劑心定，二劑火清，三劑全愈。此證切實為陽虛者，當此人素有眩暈，面色紅明，倒時額鼻有微汗，陰器欲舉，胃熱必口有穢氣，板齒燥。

Cataplexy of Yang Deficiency

People may faint all of sudden due to that the deficient heart fire cannot go down to interact with kidney, a yang deficiency case. Formula:

人參	rén shén	Root of Panax ginseng	1 liang
白朮	bái zhú	Rhizome of Atractylodes macrocephala	1 liang
生棗仁	shēng zǎo rén	Fresh seed of Ziziphus jujuba	1 liang
茯神	fú shén	Sclerotium of Poria cocos	5 qian

附子	fù zǐ	Lateral root of Aconitum carmichaeli	1 qian
甘草	gān cǎo	Root of Glycyrrhiza uralensis	1 qian
生半夏	shēng bàn xià	Unprepared rhizome of Pinellia ternata	3 qian

Upon intake, phlegm calms down and qi4 exits. The patient will be safe and sound after some continuous dosages. There are cases of sudden faint due to that stomach heat and heart fire cannot be pacified, which is yang deficiency as well. Formula:

人參	rén shén	Root of Panax ginseng	1 liang
元參	yuán shēn	Root of Scrophularia ningpoensis	1 liang
石膏	shí gāo	Gypsum	5 qian
花粉	huā fěn	Seed of Trichosanthes kirilowii	5 qian
麥冬	mài dōng	Tuber of Ophiopogon japonicus	3 qian
菖蒲	chāng pú	Rhizome of Acorus gramineus	1 qian

The first dose tranquilizes heart, the second clears away fire and the third cures. If patient's pulse is taken affirmatively to be a yang deficiency, he must have chronic dizziness, a reddish and bright complexion, insomnia with slight sweating at forehead and nose, and the genital organ is to erect. His stomach heart invariably leads to fetid mouth odor and dry incisors.

腎虛猝倒

人有口渴索引，眼紅氣喘，心脈洪大，舌不能言，不可作氣虛治。此乃腎虛之極，不能上滋於心，心火亢極，自焚悶亂，遂致身倒，有如中風者。法當補腎，而佐以清火之藥。方用水火兩治湯：

熟地、當歸、元參各壹兩，麥冬、生地、山萸、茯苓各伍錢，黃連、白芥子 、五味子各叁錢，水煎服，連服數劑而愈。

Cataplexy of Kidney Deficiency

People who feel thirsty for water has red eyes and panting, his heart pulse is surging and large, and his tongue cannot be used to talk properly. These are symptoms of utmost kidney deficiency, which cannot be treated as qi4 deficiency. Deficient kidney cannot upraise to enrich the heart and heart fire in turn is hyperactive and self-burning to cause oppressive disorder, which leads to cataplexy, a symptom similar to *wind stroke*[113]. Proper prescription is given on kidney tonification assisted by fire-clearing medicinals. The formula is *Shuihuo Liangzhi Tang* [pinyin: shuǐ huǒ liǎng zhì tāng, 水火兩治湯, Fire & Water Dual Treatment Decoction]:

熟地	shú dì	Prepared root of Rehmannia glutinosa	1 liang
當歸	dāng guī	Root of Angelica polimorpha	1 liang
元參	yuán shēn	Root of Scrophularia ningpoensis	1 liang
麥冬	mài dōng	Tuber of Ophiopogon japonicus	5 qian
生地	shēng dì	Fresh root of Rehmannia glutinosa	5 qian
山萸	shān yú	Fruit of Cornus officinalis	5 qian
茯苓	fú líng	Dried fungus of Poria cocos	5 qian
黃連	huáng lián	Rhizome of Coptis chinensis	3 qian
白芥子	bái jiè zǐ	Seed of Brassica alba	3 qian
五味子	wǔ wèi zǐ	Fruit of Schisandra chinensis	3 qian

A number of continuous doses will cure.

---

[113] *wind stroke*: sudden appearance of hemiplegia, deviated eyes and mouth, and impeded speech attributed to contraction of wind.

大怒猝倒

人有大怒跳躍，忽然臥地，兩臂抽搦，唇口歪邪，左目緊閉，此乃肝火血虛，內熱生風之症，當用八珍湯，加丹皮鉤籐山梔，若小便自遺，左關脈絃洪而數，此肝火血燥，當用六味湯，加鉤籐、 五味子、麥冬、川芎、當歸，愈後需改用補中益氣湯，加山梔、丹皮、 鉤籐，多服，如婦人得此症，則逍遙散加鉤籐及六味湯，便是治法。

Cataplexy of Tearing Rage

People, who jump and leap because of tearing rage, may suddenly lie down with convulsionary arms, deviated mouth and his tongue and left eye are tightly closed. This is a symptom of liver-fire-due blood deficiency and wind engendered by interior heat. Proper treatment is *Bazhen Tang* [pinyin: bā zhēn tāng, 八珍湯, Eight-treasure Decoction] together with **dān pí**, **gōu téng**, and **shān zhī**. If patient has enuresis and his left guan pulse string is surging and *rapid*[114], this is liver-fire-due blood dryness. Proper treatment is *Liuwei Tang* [pinyin: liù wèi tāng, 六味湯, Six-medicinal

114 *rapid pulse*: a pulse with more than five or six beats to one cycle of the physician's respiration, the same as tachycardia.

Decoction] together with **gōu téng**, **wǔ wèi zǐ**, **mài dōng**, **chuān xiōng** and **dāng guī**. Continuous dosages of *Buzhong Yiqi Tang* [pinyin: bǔ zhōng yì qì tāng, 補中益氣湯, Central Qi4 Tonification Decoction] is to be prescribed to convalescents together with **shān zhī**, **dān pí** and **gōu téng**. If the patient is a woman, *Xiaoyao Sang* [pinyin: xiāo yáo sǎn, 逍遙散, Free and Easy Powder] together with **gōu téng** and *Liuwei Tang* is the proper therapy.

中風不語

人有跌倒昏迷，或自臥而跌下床者，此皆氣虛而痰邪犯人之也，方用三生引：

人參壹兩，生半夏、生南星各叁錢，生附子壹個，水煎灌之。

此證又有因腎虛而得之者。夫腎主藏精，主下焦地道之生身，衝任二脈係焉。二脈與腎之大絡，同出於腎之下，起於胞之中，其衝脈因稱胞絡，為經脈之海，遂名海焉。其衝脈之上行者，滲諸陽，灌諸精；下行者，滲諸陰，灌諸絡，而溫肌肉，別絡結於跗，因腎虛而腎絡與胞內絕，不通於上則瘖，腎脈不上循喉嚨，挾舌本則不能言，二絡不通於下，則痱厥矣。方用地黃飲子：

熟地、巴戟、山萸、茯苓、麥冬、肉蓯蓉各壹兩，附子、菖蒲、五味子各伍錢，石斛陸錢，肉桂叁錢，薄荷、薑、棗，水煎服。

Wind Stroke with Aphasia

Patients may faint or fall down from their sleeping beds. These are all symptoms of qi4 deficiency when phlegmatic pathogens take advantage. The formula is *Sansheng Yin* [pinyin: sān shēng yǐn, 三生引, Three Lives Drink]:

人參 rén shén Root of Panax ginseng 1 liang
生半夏 bàn xià Rhizome of Pinellia ternata (raw) 3 qian
生南星 nán xīng Rhizome of Pinallia(raw) 3 qian
生附子 fù zǐ Lateral root of Aconitum carmichaeli(raw) 1 pc.

Water decoction is to be applied.

The disease may also be caused by kidney deficiency. Kidney is in charge of the hoarding of essence and the tunnels of life in lower energizer, and is the place to where the thoroughfare and conception vessels attach. The two vessels and the great collateral vessel of kidney all start from kidney and begin from the bladder. Its thoroughfare vessel is therefore called bladder collateral, the sea of meridians and collaterals, hence its name "the sea". Ascending of the thoroughfare penetrates into various yang and enrich them with essence; Descending of the thoroughfare penetrates into various yin and irrigates the collaterals and warm the flesh. Other collaterals joint at instep. For kidney deficiency, the kidney collateral has no connection to bladder and cannot upraise, which causes aphasia. Kidney meridian cannot go up to circulate the throat and control the tongue, which causes the speechless symptom of patients. That the two collaterals cannot go down causes paralytic syncope. The formula is *Dihuang Yinzi* [pinyin: dì huáng yǐn zǐ, 地黄飲子, Rehmannia Drink]:

熟地 shú dì Prepared root of Rehmannia glutinosa 1 liang
巴戟 bā jǐ Root of Morinda officinalis 1 liang
山萸 shān yú Fruit of Cornus officinalis 1 liang
茯苓 fú líng Dried fungus of Poria cocos 1 liang
麥冬 mài dōng Tuber of Ophiopogon japonicus 1 liang
肉蓯蓉 ròu cōng róng Fleshy stalk of Cistanche salsa 1 liang

附子	fù zǐ	Lateral root of Aconitum carmichaeli	5 qian
菖蒲	chāng pú	Rhizome of Acorus gramineus	5 qian
五味子	wǔ wèi zǐ	Fruit of Schisandra chinensis	5 qian
石斛	shí hú	Whole plant of Dendrobium nobile	6 qian
肉桂	ròu guì	Bark of Cinnamonum cassia	3 qian

The medicinals are decocted with **bò hé**, **jiāng**, and **zǎo**.

口眼歪邪

此證人多治木治金固是，而不知胃土之為尤切，當治胃土，且有經脈之分。《經》云：足陽明之經，急則口目為僻，眥急不能視，此胃土之經為歪邪也。又云：足陽明之脈，挾口環唇，口歪唇邪，此胃土之脈為歪邪也。二者治法，皆當用黃耆、當歸、人參、白芍、甘草、桂枝、升麻、葛根、秦艽、白芷、防風、黃柏、蘇木、紅花，水酒各半，煎微熱服，如初起有外感者，加蔥白三莖同煎，取微汗自愈。

此證又有心中虛極，不能運於口耳之間，輕則歪邪，重則不語。方用：

人參、茯苓、菖蒲、白芍各叁錢，白朮伍錢，甘草壹錢，半夏、肉桂各貳錢，當歸壹兩，水煎服。二劑愈。

又治法：令一人抱住身子，又一人抱住歪邪之耳輪，再令一人手摩其歪邪之處，至數百下，使面上火熱而後已，少頃口眼如故矣，最神效。

Deviated Eye and Mouth

Deviated eye and mouth[115] is mostly tackled through treating wood and metal by common practitioners, who have no idea that stomach earth should be their first priority. To treat stomach earth, a differentiation of meridian vessels is called for. In case of stomach meridian (ST), an urgent case is symptomized by deviated mouth and eye, canthi eyes cannot see. This is due to deviation of stomach earth's meridian. In case of stomach meridian vessel, the case is symptomized by pinched mouth and rounded lips, deviated mouth and lips. This is due to deviation of the vessel of stomach earth. Treatment for the above two cases is the decoction of:

黄耆	huáng qí	Root of Astragalus membranaceus
當歸	dāng guī	Root of Angelica polimorpha

[115] *deviated eye and mouth*: deviation of one eye and the mouth to one side with the eye unable to close and salivation from the homolateral corner of the mouth.

人參	rén shén	Root of Panax ginseng
白芍	bái sháo	Root of Paeonia lactiflora
甘草	gān cǎo	Root of Glycyrrhiza uralensis
桂枝	guì zhī	Twigs of Cinnamonum cassia
升麻	shēng má	Rhizome of Cimifuga foetida
葛根	gē gēn	Root of Pueraria lobata (Willd.)Ohwi
秦艽	qín jiāo	Root of Gentiana macrophylla Pall.
白芷	bái zhǐ	Root of Angelica dahurica
防風	fáng fēng	Root of Ledebouriella divaricata
黃柏	huáng bǎi	Bark of Phellodendron amurense
蘇木	sū mù	Wood of Caesalpinia sappan L.
紅花	hóng huā	Safflower

Medicinals are to be decocted in a mixture of water and ricewine fifty percent each. The decoction is to be taken lukewarm. For those whose onset is accompanied by external contraction, three pieces of **cōng bái** [蔥白, Stalk of Allium fistulosum] should be added for decoction. The patient cures after a slight sweating.

Some patients have utmost heart deficiency and cannot transport to mouth and ears, slight symptom of which is deviation and the serious symptom is aphasia. Formula:

人參	rén shén	Root of Panax ginseng	3 qian
茯苓	fú líng	Dried fungus of Poria cocos	3 qian
菖蒲	chāng pú	Rhizome of Acorus gramineus	3 qian
白芍	bái sháo	Root of Paeonia lactiflora	3 qian
白术	bái zhú	Rhizome of Atractylodes macrocephala	5 qian
甘草	gān cǎo	Root of Glycyrrhiza uralensis	1 qian
半夏	bàn xià	Rhizome of Pinellia ternata	2 qian
肉桂	ròu guì	Bark of Cinnamonum cassia	2 qian
當歸	dāng guī	Root of Angelica polimorpha	1 liang

In two doses patient cures. Another therapy: Have the patient's body held by one person, another person holds his deviated ears, and the third person rubs the deviated places for hundreds of times with his hands. Patient's face will be as hot as fire and then the deviation alleviates. Mouth and eyes will be as usual shortly afterwards. This is effective miraculously.

半身不遂

此證宜於心胃而調理之。蓋心為天真神機開發之本，胃是穀府，充大真氣之標。標本相得，則心膈間之膻中氣海所留宗氣盈溢，分布五臟三焦，上下中外，無不周偏。若標本相失，不能致其氣於氣海，而宗氣散矣。故分布不周於經脈則偏枯，不周於五臟則瘖，即此言之，未有不因真氣不周而病者也。法宜黃耆為君，參、歸、白芍為臣，防風、桂枝、鉤籐、竹瀝、薑、韭、葛、梨、乳汁為佐，治之而愈。若雜投乎烏、附、羌活之類，以涸營而耗衛，如此死者，醫殺人也。

Facial Hemiparalysis and Hemiplegia

This symptom should be treated by harmonizing and regulating heart and stomach. Heart is the genuine energy and root of life development, while stomach is the abode of grains where tips used for enlarging genuine qi4 is found. If both root and tips are attained, *ancestral qi4*[116] retained in chest center and Qìhǎi [氣海，CV6] is exuberant and well distributed among the five viscera and triple energizers, whether higher or lower, within or without. If the root and tip do not coordinate, and the healthy qi4 is not put in Qìhǎi,

[116] *ancestral qi4*: the combination of the essential qi4 derived from food with the air inhaled, stored in the chest, and serving as the dynamic force of blood circulation, respiration, voice, and bodily movements, the same as pectoral.

the ancestral qi4 will disperse. Therefore, if not well distributed among meridian vessels, hemiplegia befalls; Moreover, if not well distributed among the five viscera, aphasia is induced. In this sense, all diseases come from incorrectly distributed genuine qi4. Proper treatment is the monarchic use of **huáng qí**, ministered by **rén shén**, **dāng guī**, **bái sháo** and assisted by **fáng fēng**, **guì zhī** , **gōu téng**, **zhú lì**, **jiāng**, **jiǔ**, **gē**, **lí**and **rǔ zhī**. The symptom will be relieved with this prescription. If carelessly treated with medicinals like **wū fù** and **qiāng huó**, patient will have his nutrition dry up and his defense consumed. Then the doctor is to blame for patient's death.

半身不遂，口眼歪邪

方用：

人參、當歸、白朮各伍錢，黃耆壹兩，半夏、乾葛各叁錢，甘草壹錢，紅花貳錢，桂枝壹錢伍分，水二樽，薑三片，棗二枚，煎服。

此證人多用風藥治之，殊不見功，此藥調理氣血，故無不效。

此證由于血不行而又中風，若用驅風之品，偏枯則終不起矣。故當以養血和血為主，治風先治血，血行風自滅，此為的論。

Hemiplegia with Deviated Eyes and Mouth

Formula:

人參	rén shén	Root of Panax ginseng	5 qian
當歸	dāng guī	Root of Angelica polimorpha	5 qian
白术	bái zhú	Rhizome of Atractylodes macrocephala	5 qian
黃耆	huáng qí	Root of Astragalus membranaceus	1 liang
半夏	bàn xià	Rhizome of Pinellia ternata	3 qian
乾葛	gān gē	Root of Pueraria lobata	3 qian
甘草	gān cǎo	Root of Glycyrrhiza uralensis	1 qian
紅花	hóng huā	Safflower	2 qian
桂枝	guì zhī	Twigs of Cinnamonum cassia	1 qian 5 fen

Medicinals are to be decocted in two containers of water with three pieces of **jiāng** and two pieces of **zǎo**.

Medicinals for wind diseases rarely work here. However, the above formula harmonizing qi4 and blood rarely fail.

This symptom is due to improper movement of blood and wind stroke. If merely treated with wind-expelling medicinals, hemiplegia will be rooted. Therefore, the therapy shall be focused on blood nourishment and harmonization. Wind is tackled by treating blood, and wind will extinguish if blood moves. This is a precise rule.

癇症

此證忽然臥地，作牛馬豬羊之聲，吐痰如湧泉者，痰迷心竅也，蓋因寒而成，感寒而發也。方用：

人參、山藥、半夏各叁錢，白朮壹兩，茯神、薏仁各伍錢，肉桂、附子各壹錢，水煎服。又方：

人參、茯苓各壹兩，白朮伍錢，半夏、南星、附子、柴胡各壹錢，菖蒲參分，水煎服。此本治寒狂之方，治癇亦效。

Epilepsy

Patient suddenly lies down with livestock-like noises in throat and gushing phlegm. This is ascribed to the clouding of pericardium by phlegm, which is due to cold contraction. Formula：

人參	rén shén	Root of Panax ginseng	3 qian
山藥	shān yào	Root of Dioscorea opposita	3 qian
半夏	bàn xià	Rhizome of Pinellia ternata	3 qian
白术	bái zhú	Rhizome of Atractylodes macrocephala	1 liang
茯神	fú shén	Sclerotium of Poria cocos	5 qian
薏仁	yì rén	Seed kernel of Coix lachryma-jobi	5 qian
肉桂	ròu guì	Bark of Cinnamonum cassia	1 qian
附子	fù zǐ	Lateral root of Aconitum carmichaeli	1qian

Another formula:

人參	rén shén	Root of Panax ginseng	1 liang
茯苓	fú líng	Dried fungus of Poria cocos	1 liang
白术	bái zhú	Rhizome of Atractylodes macrocephala	5 qian
半夏	bàn xià	Rhizome of Pinellia ternata	1 qian
南星	nán xīng	Rhizome of Pinallia	1 qian
附子	fù zǐ	Lateral root of Aconitum carmichaeli	1 qian
柴胡	chái hú	Root of Bupleurum chinense	1 qian
菖蒲	chāng pú	Rhizome of Acorus gramineus	3 fen

Originally for treating cold psychosis, the formula is also applicable to epilepsy.

癲狂門

Chapter 5　Psychosis and Manic Psychosis

癲狂

此證多生於脾胃之虛寒，飲食入胃，不變精而變痰，痰迷心竅，遂成癲狂。苟徒治痰而不補氣，未有不死者也。方用：

人參、白芥子各伍錢，白朮壹兩，半夏三錢，陳皮、乾薑、肉桂各壹錢，甘草、菖蒲各伍分，水煎服。

如女人得此證，去肉桂加白芍、柴胡、黑梔，治之亦最神效。

Psychosis and Manic Psychosis

This syndrome is mostly due to deficiency cold of spleen-stomach. Food, upon intake, is turned not into essence but into phlegm, which clouds the pericardium and leads to psychosis or manic psychosis ultimately. If merely the phlegm is treated without qi4 tonification, patient will die unavoidably. Formula:

人參	rén shén	Root of Panax ginseng	5 qian
白芥子	bái jiè zǐ	Seed of Brassica alba	5 qian
白朮	bái zhú	Rhizome of Atractylodes macrocephala	5 qian
半夏	bàn xià	Rhizome of Pinellia ternata	3 qian
陳皮	chén pí	Peel of Citrus reticulate	1 qian
乾薑	gān jiāng	Dried Common ginger	1 qian
肉桂	ròu guì	Bark of Cinnamonum cassia	1 qian
甘草	gān cǎo	Root of Glycyrrhiza uralensis	5 fen
菖蒲	chāng pú	Rhizome of Acorus gramineus	5 fen

For female patients, the above formula added with **bái sháo**, **chái hú** and **hēi zhì** but without **ròu guì** is most miraculously effective.

發狂見鬼

此證氣虛而中痰也，宜固其正氣，而佐以化痰之品。方用：

人參、白朮各壹兩，半夏、南星各三錢，附子壹錢，水煎服。

男子補氣，女子補血。

Manic Psychosis with Illusions of Ghost

This symptom is due to phlegm stroke of qi4 deficiency. It is appropriate to fortify healthy qi4 with the assistance of phlegm-resolving medicinals. Formula:

人參	rén shén	Root of Panax ginseng	1 liang
白术	bái zhú	Rhizome of Atractylodes macrocephala	1 liang
半夏	bàn xià	Rhizome of Pinellia ternata	3 qian
南星	nán xīng	Rhizome of Pinallia	3 qian
附子	fù zǐ	Lateral root of Aconitum carmichaeli	1 qian

The formula tonifies qi4 of men and blood of women.

發狂不見鬼

此是內熱之證。方用：

人參、白芍、半夏各三錢，南星、黃連各貳錢，陳皮、甘草、白芥子各壹錢，水煎服。

Manic Psychosis without Illusions of Ghost

This is a symptom of interior heat. Formula:

人參	rén shén	Root of Panax ginseng	3 qian
白芍	bái sháo	Root of Paeonia lactiflora	3 qian

半夏	bàn xià	Rhizome of Pinellia ternata	3 qian
南星	nán xīng	Rhizome of Pinallia	2 qian
黃連	huáng lián	Rhizome of Coptis chinensis	2 qian
陳皮	chén pí	Peel of Citrus reticulata	1 qian
甘草	gān cǎo	Root of Glycyrrhiza uralensis	1 qian
白芥子	bái jiè zǐ	Seed of Brassica alba	1 qian

狂症

此證有因寒得之者，一時之狂也，可用白虎湯以瀉火。更有終年狂而不愈者，或拿刀殺人，或罵親戚，不認兒女，見水大喜，見食大惡，此乃心氣之虛，而熱邪乘之，痰氣侵之也。方用化狂丹：

人參、白朮、茯神各一兩，附子一分，半夏、兔絲子各三錢，菖蒲、甘草各一錢，水煎服。一劑狂定。

此方妙在補心脾胃三經而化其痰，不去瀉火，蓋瀉火則心氣益虛，而痰涎益盛，狂何以止乎？尤妙微用附子，引補心消痰之品直入心中，則氣易補而痰易消，又何用瀉火之多事哉？

此證因寒得之，何以用白虎湯？蓋血寒邪外逼，裹不熱泄而擾心胃，如冬傷於寒，春必病溫是也。

Manic Psychosis

This symptom may be attributed to cold. Those who go crazy momentarily is treated with *Baihu Tang* [pinyin: bái hǔ tāng, 白虎湯, White Tiger Decociton] for fire purging; Worse is the case of those who are crazy all the year round. They either attempt to kill people with a knife in hand, abuse their relatives or cannot recognize their own children; they greatly cheer up on seeing water and turn upon when seeing food. This is a case of heart qi4 deficiency taken advantage by heat pathogen and phlegm qi4. The formula is *Huakuang Dan* [pinyin: huà kuáng dān, 化狂丹, Craziness-resolving Teapills]:

人參	rén shén	Root of Panax ginseng	1 liang
白术	bái zhú	Rhizome of Atractylodes macrocephala	1 liang
茯神	fú shén	Sclerotium of Poria cocos	1 liang
附子	fù zǐ	Lateral root of Aconitum carmichaeli	1 fen
半夏	bàn xià	Rhizome of Pinellia ternata	3 qian
兔絲子	tù sī zǐ	Seed of Cuscuta chinensis	3 qian
菖蒲	chāng pú	Rhizome of Acorus gramineus	1 qian
甘草	gān cǎo	Root of Glycyrrhiza uralensis	1 qian

One dose cures.

The genius of this formula consists in its tonification of the three meridians of heart, spleen and stomach and in its phlegm resolution instead of fire purging. Since if fire is purged, the heart qi4 is more deficient and phlegm and drool is more excessive. How to stop manic psychosis in this case? More genius of the formula lies in its use of small quantity of **fù zǐ**, which conducts efficacy of the heart-tonifying and phlegm-resolving medicinals right into the heart, so that qi4 is further tonified and phlegm is further resolved. Why bother to purge fire after that?

The disease is contracted because of cold. Why *Baihu Tang* is employed? It expels cold pathogen from the blood so that the interior heat will not leak to disturb heart and stomach. If contracted with cold in winter, patient will have warm diseases in spring.

寒狂

凡發狂罵人，未渴索飲，與水不飲者，寒證之狂也。此必氣鬱不舒，怒氣未洩，其人必性情過於柔弱，不能自振者耳。宜補氣消痰。方用：

人參、茯神各一錢，白朮五錢，菖蒲三分，半夏、南星、附子、柴胡各一錢，水煎服，藥下喉，睡熟醒來，病如失也。

Cold Psychosis

Cold psychosis is symptomized with craziness, abusing people, request for drink without thirst but refuse to drink when given water. This is due to qi4 movement stagnation and constraint, and the angered qi4 can not be let out. Patient must have a very weak character that can not inspire him. Proper treatment is to tonfiy qi4 and resolve phlegm. Formula:

人參	rén shén	Root of Panax ginseng	1 qian
茯神	fú shén	Sclerotium of Poria cocos	1 qian
白朮	bái zhú	Rhizome of Atractylodes macrocephala	5 qian
菖蒲	chāng pú	Rhizome of Acorus gramineus	3 fen
半夏	bàn xià	Rhizome of Pinellia ternata	1 qian
南星	nán xīng	Rhizome of Pinallia	1 qian
附子	fù zǐ	Lateral root of Aconitum carmichaeli	1 qian
柴胡	chái hú	Root of Bupleurum chinense	1 qian

Upon intake of the decoction, patient will feel the disease is gone after a sound sleep.

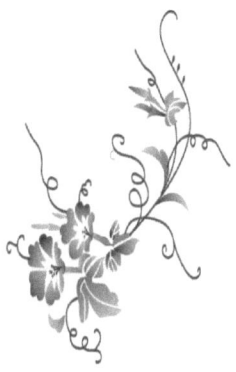

怔忡驚悸門

Chapter 6

Fearful Throbbing and Fright Palpitations

怔忡不寐

此證心經血虛也。方用：

人參、當歸、茯苓各叁錢，丹皮、麥冬各貳錢，甘草、菖蒲、五味子各壹錢，生棗仁、熟棗仁各伍錢，水煎服。

此方妙在用生、熟棗仁，生使其日間不臥，熟使其夜間不醒，又以補心之藥為佐，而怔忡安矣。

Fearful Throbbing with Insomnia

The symptom of *fearful throbbing*[117] with insomnia is ascribed to the blood deficiency of heart meridian (HT). Formula:

人參 rén shén Root of Panax ginseng 3 qian

當歸 dāng guī Root of Angelica polimorpha 3 qian

[117] *fearful throbbing*: a severe case of palpitation.

茯苓 fú líng Dried fungus of Poria cocos 3 qian

丹皮 dān pí Bark of the root of Paeonia suffruticosa 2 qian

麥冬 mài dōng Tuber of Ophiopogon japonicus 2 qian

甘草 gān cǎo Root of Glycyrrhiza uralensis 1 qian

菖蒲 chāng pú Rhizome of Acorus gramineus 1 qian

五味子 wǔ wèi zǐ Fruit of Schisandra chinensis 1 qian

生棗仁 shēng zǎo rén Fresh seed of Ziziphus jujuba 5 qian

熟棗仁 shú zǎo rén Prepared seed of Ziziphus jujuba 5 qian

The genius of this formula consists in its employment of **shēng zǎo rén** and **shú zǎo rén**. **Shēng zǎo rén** keeps the patient awake during the day while **shú zǎo rén** gives him a sound sleep during the night. With the assistance of these heart tonifying medicinals, fearful throbbing will be settled.

心驚不安夜臥不睡

此心病而實腎病也，宜心腎兼治。方用：

人參、茯苓、茯神、熟地、山萸、當歸各參兩，遠志貳兩，菖蒲叁錢，黃連、肉桂、砂仁各伍錢，生棗仁、白芥子各壹兩，麥冬參兩，蜜丸。每日下五錢，湯酒俱可。

此方治心驚不安與不寐耳。用人參、當歸、茯神、麥冬足矣，即為起火不寐，亦不過用黃連足矣，何以反用熟地、山萸補腎之藥，又加肉桂以助火？不知人之心驚，乃腎氣不入於心也；不寐乃心氣不歸於腎也。今用熟地山萸補腎，則腎氣可通於心。肉桂以補命門之火，則腎氣既溫，相火有救，君火相得，自然上下同心，君臣合德矣。然補腎固是，而亦有肝氣不上於心而成此證者，如果有之，宜再加白芍二兩，兼補肝木，斯心泰然矣。

Palpitations with Insomniac Nights

This is a syndrome that heart disease develops excessively into a kidney disease. The therapy is dual treatment of both heart and kidney. Formula:

人參	rén shén	Root of Panax ginseng	3 liang
茯苓	fú líng	Dried fungus of Poria cocos	3 liang
茯神	fú shén	Sclerotium of Poria cocos	3 liang
熟地	shú dì	Prepared root of Rehmannia glutinosa	3 liang
山萸	shān yú	Fruit of Cornus officinalis	3 liang
當歸	dāng guī	Root of Angelica polimorpha	3 liang

遠志	yuǎn zhì	Root of Polygala tenuifolia	2 liang
菖蒲	chāng pú	Rhizome of Acorus gramineus	3 qian
黄連	huáng lián	Rhizome of Coptis chinensis	5 qian
肉桂	ròu guì	Bark of Cinnamonum cassia	5 qian
砂仁	shā rén	Fruit of Amomum villosum	5 qian
生棗仁	shēng zǎo rén	Fresh seed of Ziziphus jujuba	1 liang
白芥子	bái jiè zǐ	Seed of Brassica alba	1 liang
麥冬	mài dōng	Tuber of Ophiopogon japonicus	3 liang

Honeyed pills of five qian per day shall be taken with either hot water or wine.

For treating palpitations with insomnia, medicinals of **rén shén**, **dāng guī**, **fú shén** and **mài dōng** are enough in the formula. Even in case of insomnia of fire flaming, it is enough to employ **huáng lián** to deal with. Why kidney-tonifying medicinals of **shú dì** and **shān yú** are employed with assistance of **ròu guì** to help with the fire in this formula? It is rarely known that palpitation is ascribed to kidney qi4's failure to enter the heart and insomnia is traced to heart qi4's failure to return to kidney. Here, we use **shú dì** and **shān yú** for kidney tonification, kidney qi4 can join with the heart in this way; we use **ròu guì** to tonfiy life gate fire, so that kidney qi4 is warmed, ministerial fire get its right and the monarch and fire coordinates, hence the result of coordination of both the upper and the lower and cooperation between monarch and ministers. Aside from kidney tonification, there are cases resulted from liver qi4's failure to upraise into heart. In this case, additional two liang of **bái sháo** is recommended for liver wood tonification, the heart will be settled down then.

恐怕

人夜臥交睫，則夢爭鬥負敗，恐怖之狀，難以形容。人以為心病，誰知是肝病乎？蓋肝藏魂，肝血虛則魂失養，故交睫若魘。此乃肝膽虛怯，故負恐維多。此非火補，不克奏功；而草木之品，不堪任重，當以酒化鹿角膠，空腹服之可愈。蓋鹿角膠大補精血，血旺則神自安矣。

何以知肝氣不上于心，此人當面色青，或潮熱，或手足燒，或眩暈左俋漲。

Frightful Palpitations

Some patients, upon closing their eyes in the night, dream of fighting with others and failures of fighting, and it is hard to describe the horrible appearances on their faces. Normally taken as a heart disease, *frightful palpitations*[118] are rarely known as a liver one. Liver is the abode of *ethereal soul*[119], which will not be properly nourished if liver blood is in deficiency, from whence the nightmare, a result of deficient timidity of liver and gallbladder. It cannot be treated but with great tonification. However, herbs cannot be assigned with this task. The proper therapy is to dissolve **lù jiǎo jiāo** in wine and to take when with empty stomach. **Lù jiǎo jiāo** greatly tonifies essence and blood, the *ethereal soul* is then calmed once the blood is exuberant.

How do we know the liver qi4 fails to upraise into heart? Patient must have a bluish complexion, *tidal fever*[120] or fevered extremities, dizziness or distension of left abdomen.

---

[118] *fright palpitations:* palpitation ascribed to being frightened.

[119] *ethereal soul*: the moral and spiritual part of the human being.

[120] *tidal fever*: fever with periodic rise and fall of body temperature at fixed hours of the day like the morning and evening tides.

神氣不寧

人有每臥則魂飛揚，覺身在床而魂離體矣。驚悸多魘，通夕不寐，人皆以為心病也，誰知是肝經受邪乎？蓋肝氣一虛，邪氣襲之；肝藏魂，肝受邪，魂無依，是以魂飛揚而若離體也。法用珍珠母為君，龍齒佐之。珍珠母入肝為第一，龍齒與肝同類，龍齒虎睛，今人例以為鎮心之藥，詎知龍齒安魂，虎睛定魄。東方蒼龍，木也，屬肝而藏魂；西方白虎，金也，屬肺而藏魄。龍能變化，故魂游而不定；虎能專靜，故魄止而有守，是以治魄不寧宜虎睛，治魂飛揚宜龍齒，藥各有當也。此證岳每用桂枝湯溫膽湯參之頗效。

Disorder of Spiritual Qi4

Whenever touching his pillow, patient feels his soul lifted while only his body is left on bed. He has fright palpitations and nightmares, and is sleepless throughout the night. Normally regarded as heart disease, this symptom is in fact due to pathogen-affected liver meridian (LR), since once liver qi4 is in deficiency, pathogens will take advantage. Liver holds the soul, if liver is affected by pathogens, the soul finds nowhere to attach to. Therefore, patient feels his soul lifted as if leaving his body. The proper therapy is to use **zhēn zhū mŭ** as monarch with assistance of **lóng chĭ**. **Zhēn zhū mŭ** enters the liver at first, and **lóng chĭ** is the same as liver in nature. **Lóng chĭ** and **hŭ jīng** are customarily regarded as heart-calming medicinals, but it is rarely known that **lóng chĭ** settles the soul and **hŭ jīng** calms the soul. Green dragon of the East is wood, it belongs to liver in property and hides the *ethereal soul*; White tiger of the West is metal, it belongs to lung in property and hides the *corporal soul*[121]. The dragon is capable of changes so that *ethereal soul* reaches far away; tigers are good at couching so that *corporal soul* adheres and stays. Therefore, for treating uneasiness of *corporal soul* **hŭ jīng** is used, and for treating uneasiness of *ethereal soul* **lóng chĭ** is applied. Medicinals have their own usages.

Yue often used *Guizhi Tang* [pinyin: guì zhī tāng, 桂枝湯, Cassia Twig Decoction] and *Wendan Tang* [pinyin: wēn dăn tāng, 溫膽湯, Gall Bladder Warming Decoction] as a combined medicament, which is quite effective.

---

[121] *corporal soul*: the animating part of one's mind.

腰腿肩背手足疼痛門

Chapter 7

Pains in Waist, Legs, Shoulders, Back and Extremities

滿身皆痛

手足心腹一身皆痛，將治手乎？治足乎？治肝為主，蓋肝氣一舒，諸痛自愈。不可頭痛救頭、足痛救足也。方用：

柴胡、甘草、陳皮、梔子各壹錢，白芍、薏仁、茯苓各伍錢，當歸、蒼朮各貳錢，水煎服。

此逍遙散之變化也，舒肝而又去溼去火，治一經而諸經無不愈也。

Overall Pain

How to deal with an overall pain in the extremities, heart and abdomen? To treat the hands, or to treat the feet? We should chiefly treat the liver, since once liver qi4 is relaxed all pains will be cured. We should not treat the head when head aches and treat the feet when feet pain. Formula:

柴胡	chái hú	Root of Bupleurum chinense	1 qian
甘草	gān cǎo	Root of Glycyrrhiza uralensis	1 qian
陳皮	chén pí	Peel of Citrus reticulata	1qian
梔子	zhī zǐ	Fruit of Gardenia jasminoides	1 qian
白芍	bái sháo	Root of Paeonia lactiflora	5 qian
薏仁	yì rén	Seed kernel of Coix lachryma-jobi	5 qian
茯苓	fú líng	Dried fungus of Poria cocos	5 qian
當歸	dāng guī	Root of Angelica polimorpha	2 qian
蒼朮	cāng zhú	Rhizome of Swordlike Atractylodes	2 qian

This is an adjusted formula of *Xiaoyao San* [pinyin: xiāo yáo sǎn, 逍遙散, Free and Easy Powder], which soothes the liver, dispels dampness and fire, and cures all meridians through treating just one of them.

腰痛

痛而不能俯者，溼氣也。方用：

柴胡、澤瀉、豬苓、白芥子各壹錢，防已貳錢，白朮、甘草各伍錢，肉桂參分，山藥叁錢，水煎服。

此方妙在入腎去溼，不是入腎而補水。初痛者，一、二劑可以奏功，日久必多服為妙。

Lumbago

Sufferers from lumbago cannot stoop. The symptom is due to dampness. Formula:

柴胡	chái hú	Root of Bupleurum chinense	1 qian
澤瀉	zé xiè	Rhizome of Alisma plantago-aquatica	1 qian
豬苓	zhū líng	Agaric	1 qian
白芥子	bái jiè zǐ	Seed of Brassica alba	1 qian
防己	fáng jǐ	Root of Aristolochia fangchi	2 qian
白术	bái zhú	Rhizome of Atractylodes macrocephala	5 qian
甘草	gān cǎo	Root of Glycyrrhiza uralensis	5 qian
肉桂	ròu guì	Bark of Cinnamonum cassia	3 fen
山藥	shān yào	Root of Dioscorea opposite	3 qian

The genius of this formula lies in its entering kidney to dispel dampness instead of entering kidney to tonfiy water. One or two doses for incipient sufferers are just enough, but more doses are recommended for chronic sufferers.

腰痛

痛而不能直者，風寒也。方用逍遙散加防已一錢，一劑可愈。若日久者，當加杜仲一兩，改白朮二錢，酒煎服。

十劑而愈。又方：

杜仲壹兩鹽炒，破故紙伍錢鹽炒，熟地、白朮各參兩，核桃仁貳錢，蜜丸。每日空心白水送下五錢。服完可愈，如未全愈，再服一料，必愈。

Lumbago

Lumbago with symptom of inability to strengthen one's back is due to wind-cold, and the formula is *Xiaoyao San* [pinyin: xiāo yáo sǎn, 逍遙散, Free and Easy Powder] added with one qian of **fáng jǐ**. One dose cures. Chronic sufferers may be treated with additional one liang of **dù zhòng** and two qian of **gǎi bái zhú**. The medicinals are decocted in wine and it cures in ten doses. Another formula:

杜仲鹽炒 dù zhòng Bark of Eucommia ulmoidis (salt fried) 1 liang

破故紙鹽炒 pò gù zhǐ Foliage of Clammy Hopseedbush (salt fried) 5 qian

熟地 shúdì Prepared root of Rehmannia glutinosa 3 liang

白朮 bái zhú Rhizome of Atractylodes macrocephala 3 liang

核桃仁 táo rén Seed of Prunus persica 2 qian

Five qian of honeyed pills are taken everyday with boiled water when stomach is empty. It cures after taking the dosage, otherwise another dose is needed. The second will surely cure.

腰痛

凡痛而不止者，腎經之病，乃脾溼之故。方用：

白朮肆兩，薏仁參兩，芡實貳兩，水六碗，煎一碗，一氣飲之。此方治夢遺之病亦神效。

Lumbago

Lumbago with incessant pain is due to sickness of kidney meridian (KI) for spleen dampness. Formula:

白朮 bái zhú Rhizome of Atractylodes macrocephala 4 liang
薏仁 yì rén Seed kernel of Coix lachryma-jobi 3 liang
芡實 qiàn shí Seed of Euryale ferox 2 liang

Six bowls of water is decocted into one bowl of decoction for drinking at one draft. This formula is miraculously effective to dream emission as well.

腰腿筋骨痛

方用養血湯：

當歸、生地、肉桂、牛膝、杜仲、破故紙、茯苓、防風各壹錢，川芎五分，甘草參分，核桃貳個，山萸、土茯苓各貳錢，水酒煎服。

Painful Sinews and Bones of Waist and Legs

The prescription is *Yangxue Tang* [pinyin: yǎng xuè tāng, 養血湯, Blood-nourishing Decoction]:

當歸	dāng guī	Root of Angelica polimorpha	1 qian
生地	shēng dì	Root of Rehmannia glutinosa Libosch.	1 qian
肉桂	ròu guì	Bark of Cinnamonum cassia	1 qian
牛膝	niú xī	Root of Achyranthes bidentata	1 qian
杜仲	dù zhòng	Bark of Eucommia ulmoidis	1 qian
破故紙	pò gù zhǐ	Foliage of Clammy Hopseedbush	1 qian
茯苓	fú líng	Dried fungus of Poria cocos	1 qian
防風	fáng fēng	Root of Ledebouriella divaricata	1 qian
川芎	chuān xiōng	Root of Ligusticum wallichii	5 fen
甘草	gān cǎo	Root of Glycyrrhiza uralensis	3 fen
核桃	hé tao	Walnut seed	2 pcs.

山萸	shān yú	Fruit of Cornus officinalis	2 qian
土茯苓	fú líng	Dried fungus of Poria cocos	2 qian

The medicinals should be decocted in wine.

腰痛足亦痛

方用：

黃耆半斤，防風、茯苓各伍錢，薏仁伍兩，杜仲壹兩，肉桂壹錢，車前子叁錢，水十碗，煎二碗，入酒，以醉為主，醒即愈。

腰足痛，明係是腎虛而氣衰，更加之溼，自必作楚。妙在不補腎而單益氣，蓋氣足則血生，血生則邪退；又助之薏仁、茯苓、車前之類去溼，溼去而血活矣。況又有杜仲之健腎、肉桂之溫腎、防風之蕩風乎！

Lumbago with Podalgia

Formula:

黃耆	huáng qí	Root of Astragalus membranaceus	half jin
防風	fáng fēng	Root of Ledebouriella divaricata	5 qian
茯苓	fú líng	Dried fungus of Poria cocos	5 qian
薏仁	yì rén	Seed kernel of Coix lachryma-jobi	5 liang

杜仲	dù zhòng	Bark of Eucommia ulmoidis	1 liang
肉桂	ròu guì	Bark ofCinnamonum cassia	1 qian
車前子	chē qián zǐ	Seed of Plantago asiatica	3 qian

Ten bowls of water is to be decocted into two bowls of decoction and mixed with wine. Patient shall be drunk upon intake, and the cure is attained after the patient wakes up.

Lumbago with podalgia is obviously a symptom of kidney deficiency of qi4 debilitation. With dampness, it certainly hurts. The genius of the formula consists in its sole qi4 tonification instead of kidney tonification, since when qi4 is enough blood is engendered, which drives back pathogens and help with dispelling pathogens with assistance of medicinals like **yì rén**, **fú ling**, and **chē qián zǐ**. Blood is activated once the dampness is dispelled, let along the kidney fortification effecacy of **dù zhòng**, kidney warming efficacy of **ròu guì** and wind cleansing of **fáng fēng**.

腿痛

身不離床褥，傴僂之狀可掬，乃寒溼之氣侵也。方用：

白朮伍錢，芡實貳錢，肉桂壹錢，茯苓、萆薢各壹兩，杜仲叁錢 薏仁貳兩。水煎，日日服之，不必改方，久之自奏大功。

Skelalgia

Patient is bed-bond with a humpbacked figure. This is due to invasion of cold and dampness. Formula:

白朮 bái zhúRhizome of Atractylodes macrocephala 5 qian
芡實 qiàn shí Seed of Euryale ferox 2 qian
肉桂 ròu guì Bark of Cinnamonum cassia 1 qian
茯苓 fú líng Dried fungus of Poria cocos 1 liang
萆薢 bì xiè Rhizome of Dioscorea hypoglauca 1 liang
杜仲 dù zhòng Bark of Eucommia ulmoidis 3 qian
薏仁 yì rén Seed kernel of Coix lachryma-jobi 2 liang

The decoction is to be taken daily. This formula does not need any adjustment and it cures if given enough time.

兩臂肩膊痛

此手經之病，肝氣之鬱也。方用：

當歸、白芍各參兩，柴胡、陳皮各伍錢，羌活、秦艽、白芥子、半夏各叁錢，附子壹錢，水六碗，煎三沸，取汁一碗，入黃酒服之，一醉而愈。

此方妙在用白芍為君，以平肝木，不來侮胃；而羌活、柴胡又去風，直走手經之上；秦艽亦是風藥；而兼附子攻邪，邪自退出；半夏、陳皮、白芥子為祛痰聖藥，風邪去而痰不留；更得附子無經不達，而其痛如失也。

Pain in the Arms and Shoulders

This is a disease of hand meridian, and the depression of liver qi4. Formula:

當歸	dāng guī	Root of Angelica polimorpha	3 liang
白芍	bái sháo	Root of Paeonia lactiflora	3 liang
柴胡	chái hú	Root of Bupleurum chinense	5 qian
陳皮	chén pí	Dried peel of Citrus reticulata	5 qian
羌活	qiāng huó	Rhizome of Notopterygium forbesii Boiss.	3 qian
秦艽	qín jiāo	Root of Gentiana macrophylla Pall.	3 qian
白芥子	bái jiè zǐ	Seed of Brassica alba	3 qian
半夏	bàn xià	Rhizome of Pinellia ternata	3 qian

附子 fù zǐ Lateral root of Aconitum carmichaeli 1 qian

Six bowls of water is decocted with the medicinals. After three times of boiling, take one bowl of decoction with rice wine. It cures after inebriation.

The beauty of this formula consists in its monarchic use of **bái sháo**, which soothes liver wood but without insulting stomach. Moreover, **qiāng huó** and **chái hú** dispels wind and the efficacy of them goes upward along the lung meridian. **Qín jiāo** is also a wind medicinal and **fù zǐ** forces pathogens to retreat. **Bàn xià**, **chén pí**, and **bái jiè zǐ** are miraculous medicinals for dispelling phlegm which cannot stay after the wind is gone. Furthermore, there is no meridian that efficacy of **fù zǐ** can not reach. The pain will be as if gone.

手足痛

手足，肝之分野，而人乃為脾經之熱，不知散肝木之鬱結，而手足之痛自去。方用逍遙散加梔子叁錢，半夏貳錢，白芥子貳錢，水煎服。二劑，其痛如失。

蓋肝木作祟，脾不敢當其鋒，氣散於四肢，結而不伸，所以作楚，今平其肝氣，則脾氣自舒矣。

Chiropodalgia

The extremities are affiliated to liver. However, people think it is due to heat of spleen meridian (SP). They do not know if liver wood depression is dispersed, chiropodalgia will be gone by itself. The formula is *Xiaoyao San* [pinyin: xiāo yáo sǎn, 逍遙散, Free and Easy Powder] added with three qian of **zhī zǐ**, two qian of **bàn xià** and two qian of **bái jiè zǐ**.

The pain will be as if gone in two doses. This symptom is ascribed to troubles of liver wood which is not refrained by the spleen. As a result, qi4 disperses to the extremities and bonds, and hence the pains. Now liver qi4 is normalized and the spleen qi4 will be soothed.

胸背手足頸項腰膝痛

筋骨牽引，坐臥不得，時時走易不定，此是痰涎伏在心膈上下。或令人頭痛，夜間喉中如鋸聲，口流涎唾，手足重，腿冷，治法用控涎丹，不足十劑其病如失矣。

Pains in Chest, Back, Extremities, Neck, Nape, Waist and Knees

Sinews and bones are felt stretched; patients are restless

and walk constantly. This is clouding of drool on the pericardium, which makes patient either have headache, spittle runs down from mouth, or have heavy extremities, cold legs or grunting with noises like a wood saw working during the night. The proper therapty is *Kongyan Dan* [pinyin: kòng yán dān, 控涎丹, Drool-controlling Teapills]. The disease will be as if gone in ten doses.

背骨痛

此證乃腎水衰耗，不能上潤於腦，則河車之路，乾澀而難行，故作痛也。方用：

黃耆、熟地各壹兩，山萸肆錢，白朮、防風各伍錢，五味子壹錢，茯苓叁錢，附子壹分，麥冬貳錢，水煎服。

此方補氣補水，去溼去風，潤筋滋骨，何痛之不愈哉？

此方補氣補水，去溼去風，潤筋滋骨，何痛之不愈哉。

Pains in Backbone

This symptom is caused by the exhaustion of kidney water that cannot upraise to moisten brain. The channel for the *river vehicle*[122] is dry and hard, hence the pain. Formula:

---

[122] *river vehicle*: an alternate name for kidney.

黃耆 huáng qí Root of Astragalus membranaceus 1 liang
熟地 shú dì Prepared Rroot of Rehmannia glutinosa1 liang
山萸 shān yú Fruit of Cornus officinalis 4 qian
白术 bái zhú Rhizome of Atractylodes macrocephala 5 qian
防風 fáng fēng Root of Ledebouriella divaricata 5 qian
五味子 wǔ wèi zǐ Fruit of Schisandra chinensis 1 qian
茯苓 fú líng Dried fungus of Poria cocos 3 qian
附子 fù zǐ Lateral root of Aconitum carmichaeli 1 fen
麥冬 mài dōng Tuber of Ophiopogon japonicus 2 qian

This formula tonifies qi4 and water, dispels dampness and wind, and it moistens sinews and nourishes bone. How can the pain stay?

腰痛兼頭痛

上下相殊也，如何治之乎？治腰乎？治頭乎？誰知是腎氣不通乎。蓋腎氣上通於腦，而腦氣下達於腎，上下雖殊，而氣實相通。法當用溫補之藥，以火益其腎中之陰，則上下之氣通矣。方用：

熟地壹兩，杜仲、麥冬各伍錢，五味子貳錢，水煎服。

一劑即愈。

方內熟地、杜仲，腎中藥也，腰痛是其專功。今並頭而亦愈者何也？蓋此頭痛，是腎氣不上達之故，用補腎之味，則腎氣旺而上通於腦，故腰不痛而頭亦不痛矣。

Simultaneous Lumbago and Headache

The upper and the lower body are greatly different, how can they be treated both? To treat the waist? Or to treat the head? Who knows it is actually due to blockage of kidney qi4? Kidney qi4 upraises to join with the brain, and brain qi4 goes down to reach the kidney. Though far detached, they are in reality connected by qi4. A proper therapy is the employment of warm-tonifying medicinals that benefits greatly the kidney yin, so that upper and lower qi4 joints. Formula:

熟地 shú dì Prepared Rroot of Rehmannia glutinosa 1 liang
杜仲 dù zhòng Bark of Eucommia ulmoidis 5 qian
麥冬 mài dōng Tuber of Ophiopogon japonicus 5 qian
五味子 wǔ wèi zǐ Fruit of Schisandra chinensis 2 qian

One dose cures. **Shú dì** and **dù zhòng**, two medicinals for kidney specify in treating lumbago. Why is the headache cured as well? This headache is due to failure of kidney qi4 to upraise and joint. With kidney-tonifying medicinals, kidney qi4 flourishes to joint with the brain. Lumbago and headache are therefore cured together.

心腹痛門

Chapter 8 Heart and Abdominal Pain

心痛辨

心痛之證有二，一則寒氣侵心而痛，一則火氣焚心而痛。寒氣侵心者，手足反溫；火氣焚心者，手足反冷，以此辨之最得。

寒痛方用：良薑、白朮、草烏、貫仲各叁錢，肉桂、甘草各壹錢，水煎服。

熱痛方用：黑梔叁錢，白朮伍錢，甘草、半夏、柴胡各壹錢，水煎服。

心不可使痛，或寒或火，皆沖心包耳。

Differentiation on Heart Pain

There are two types of *heart pain*[123], one is pain of cold qi4's invasion of heart, and the other is pain of fire qi4's burning of heart. For the former, patients have warm extremities, while for the latter, patients have cold ones. This

[123] *heart pain*: a general term for pain in the precordial and epigastric regions.

is the most useful way of differentiation.

The formula for cold pain:

良薑 liáng jiāng Rhizome Alpinia officinarum Hance 3 qian
白术 bái zhú Rhizome of Atractylodes macrocephala 3 qian
草烏 cǎo wū Root of Vilmorin Monkshood 3 qian
貫仲 guàn zhòng Rhizome of Aspidium crassirhizoma 3 qian
肉桂 ròu guì Bark of Cinnamonum cassia 1 qian
甘草 gān cǎo Root of Glycyrrhiza uralensis 1 qian

The formula for heat pain:

黑梔 hēi zhì Fruit or root of Gardenia stenphylla Merr.3 qian
白术 bái zhú Rhizome of Atractylodes macrocephala 5 qian
甘草 gān cǎo Root of Glycyrrhiza uralensis 1 qian
半夏 bàn xià Rhizome of Pinellia ternata 1 qian
柴胡 chái hú Root of Bupleurum chinense 1 qian

Treatment of the heart pain shall not be delayed. Either cold or heat, they both assault the pericardium.

久病心痛

心乃神明之君，一毫邪氣不可干犯，犯則立死。經年累月而痛者，邪氣犯心包絡也。但邪有寒熱之辨，如惡寒見水如仇，火熨之則快，此寒邪也。方用：

蒼朮貳錢，白朮伍錢，當歸壹兩，肉桂、良薑各壹錢，水煎服。

如見水喜悅，手按之而轉痛者，熱氣犯心包絡也。方用：

白芍壹兩，黑梔、當歸、生地各叁錢，甘草壹錢，陳皮捌分，水煎服。

寒熱二證，皆責之於肝也。肝屬木，心屬火，木衰不能生火，則包絡寒，補肝而邪自退。若包絡之熱，由於肝經之熱，瀉肝而火自消也。

心腹之痛共有九種，其實皆心包絡、胃脘、膻中及腹痛，無真心痛也，蟲痛、注痛、氣痛、血痛、悸痛、食痛、飲痛、冷痛、熱痛、證各有辨，其用藥亦大有不同，如蟲痛則唇上有瘡，痛時作時止，可與烏梅圓，注痛則兼頭痛，或抽慉或妄語，可與蘇合丸，氣痛則或上或下，或前或後，有肝、有胃、有肺，可與左金丸、平胃散之屬，血痛則有痞塊，可與桃仁湯、失笑散，悸痛則按之不拒，可與理中湯、妙香散，食痛則拒按發熱，可與承氣湯、檳榔丸，飲痛則吐清水，俹下有水聲，可與二陳湯，甚者十棗湯，冷痛熱痛則此二方可用，先生此書因窮鄉僻壤而設，執此可以應急，且免誤於庸醫，故去煩就簡也。

Heart Pain of Chronic Diseases

Heart is the monarch of spiritual mind and shall not be invaded even for the tiniest bit. Otherwise patient dies instantly. Chronic heart pain is ascribed to pathogenic invasion of pericardium. However, pathogens are of cold or heat property. If with aversion to cold, patient abhors seeing water and is much relieved with a hot object applied to chest, it is cold pathogen. Formula:

蒼朮 cāng zhú Rhizome of Swordlike Atractylodes 2 qian
白术 bái zhúRhizome of Atractylodes macrocephala 5 qian
當歸 dāng guī Root of Angelica polimorpha 1 liang
肉桂 ròu guì Bark of Cinnamonum cassia 1 qian
良薑 liáng jiāng Rhizome Alpinia officinarum Hance 1 qian

If the patient lightens to see water and his heart pains if pressed, it is invasion of pericardium by heat qi4. Formula:

白芍 bái sháo Root of Paeonia lactiflora 1 liang
黑栀 hēi zhì Fruit or root of Gardenia stenphylla Merr. 3qian
當歸 dāng guī Root of Angelica polimorpha qian
生地 shēng dì Fresh root of Rehmannia glutinosa 3 qian
甘草 gān cǎo Root of Glycyrrhiza uralensis 1 qian

陳皮	chén pí	Peel of Citrus reticulata	8 fen

Liver is to blame for either heat or cold pain. Liver is wood in property and heart is fire. If wood declines, the fire will not be lighted to warm pericardium. If liver is tonified, pathogens will retreat. If heat of pericardium is due to heat of liver meridian, the fire will be extinguished once liver is purged.

There are a total nine types of heart pain, which are in fact pains of pericardium, *stomach duct*[124], chest center and abdomen and none of these is true heart pain. Parasitogenic abdominal pain, energizer pain, qi4 pain, blood pain, palpitation pain, food pain, drink pain, cold pain and heat pain, all syndromes shall be differentiated and medicated in different ways. For instance, parasitogenic abdominal pain, with symptoms of lip sore that constantly pains, can be treated with ***wū méi yuán***; Energizer pain, accompanied by headache, convulsion or paraphasia can be treated with *Suhe Wan* [pinyin: sū hé wán, 蘇合丸, Storax Bolus]; Qi4 pain, either up or down, back and forth with variation of liver qi4

124 *stomach duct*: stomach duct refers to (1) stomach cavity and adjoining section of theesophagus; (2) epigastrium.

pain, stomach qi4 pain and lung qi4 pain, can be treated with medicines like *Zuojin Wan* [pinyin: zuǒ jīn wán, 左金丸, Left Gold Bolus] and *Pingwei San* [pinyin: ping wèi sǎn, 平胃散, Stomach-soothing Powder]; Blood pain with *stuffiness*[125] lump can be treated with *Taoren Tang* [pinyin: táo rén tāng, 桃仁湯, Semen Persicae Decoction] and *Shixiao San* [pinyin: shī xiào sǎn, 失笑散, Wonderful Powder for Relieving Blood Stagnation]; Patient with palpitation pain can not resist oppression, and shall be treated with *Lizhong Tang* [pinyin: lǐ zhōng tāng, 理中湯, Decoction for Mid Energizer Regulation] or *Miaoxiang San* [pinyin: miào xiāng sǎn, 妙香散, Miraculously Fragrant Powder]; Patient with food pain is afraid of oppression and has heat, they can be treated with *Chengqi4 Tang* [pinyin: chéng qì tāng, 承氣湯, Qi4-restoring Decoction] or *Binlang Wan* [pinyin: bīng lang wán, 檳榔丸, Betelnut Bolus]; Drink pain has symptoms of vomiting of clear water and rumbling noise of water in abdomen, it can be treated with E*rchen Tang* [pinyin: èr chén tāng, 二陳湯, Two Old Medicinals Decoction] or *Shizao Tang* [pinyin: shí zǎo tāng, 十棗湯,

125 *stuffiness*: a localized subjective feeling of fullness and blockage.

Ten Jujube Decoction]. These two formulae are also applicable to cold pain and heat pain. The author intentionally adjusted formulae for those remote hinterlands with simplification of literary writing by leaving out superfluous words so as to be more applicable for emergency and to avoid mal-treatment of those charlatans.

腹痛

痛不可忍，按之愈痛，口渴飲以涼水，則痛少止，少頃依然大痛。此火結在大小腸也，若不急治，一時氣絕。方用定痛如神湯：

黑梔、蒼朮各叁錢，甘草、厚樸各壹錢，茯苓壹兩，白芍伍錢，水煎服。

此方舒肝經之氣，利膀胱之水，瀉水逐瘀。再加大黃壹錢，水煎服，勿遲。

Abdominal Pain

Abdominal pain[126] is irresistible and becomes worse if pressed. Patient feels thirsty and the pain relieves a little

126 *abdominal pain:* pain in the region between the hypochondrium and pubic hairline.

after drinking cold water, but bounces back after a while. This is fire stagnation at large and small intestines. If not treated instantly, patient may lose breath in a while. The formula is *Dingtong Rushen Tang* [pinyin: dìng tòng rú shén tāng, 定痛如神湯, Miraculous Pain-relieving Decoction]:

黑栀	hēi zhì	Fruit or root of Gardenia stenphylla Merr.	3 qian
蒼朮	cāng zhú	Rhizome of Swordlike Atractylodes	3 qian
甘草	gān căo	Root of Glycyrrhiza uralensis	1 qian
厚樸	hòu pò	Bark of Magnolia officinalis	1 qian
茯苓	fú líng	Dried fungus of Poria cocos	1 liang
白芍	bái sháo	Root of Paeonia lactiflora	5 qian

This formula relaxes qi4 of liver meridian, induces water of bladder, purges water and expels stasis. If with additional one qian of **dà huáng**, the decoction should be taken with no delay.

腹痛

腸中有痞塊，一時發作，而痛不可手按者。方用：白朮貳兩，枳實壹兩，馬糞炒焦伍錢，好酒煎服。冷氣心腹痛，方用火龍丹：

硫磺醋製壹兩，胡椒壹錢，白礬肆錢，醋打蕎麵為丸，如桐子大。每服二十五丸，米湯下。

Abdominal Pain

A formula for those with abdominal stuffiness lump and irresistible to oppression once the pain attacks:

白术	bái zhú	Rhizome of Atractylodes macrocephala	2 liang
枳實	zhǐ shí	Unripe fruit of Poncirus trifoliata	1 liang
馬糞	mǎ fèn	Horse manure (parched)	5 qian

The medicinals are decocted in good wine. For cold qi4 heart and abdominal pain, the prescription is *Huolong Dan* [pinyin: huǒ long dān, 火龍丹, Fire Dragon Pill]:

硫磺醋製	liú huáng	Sulphur prepared with vinegar	1 liang
胡椒	hú jiāo	Pepper	1 qian
白礬	bái fán	Alunite	4 qian

Mixed with vinegar and buckwheat flour, medicinals are processed into pills in size of tung-oil tree seed to be taken with thin rice soup twenty-five pills each time.

胃氣痛

人病不能飲食，或食而不化，作痛作滿，或兼吐瀉，此肝木剋脾土也。方用：

白芍、當歸、柴胡、茯苓各貳錢，白朮叁錢，甘草、白芥子各壹錢，水煎服。

有火加梔子貳錢；無火加肉桂壹錢；有食加山查叁錢；傷麵食加枳殼壹錢、麥芽壹錢；有痰加半夏壹錢。有火能散，有寒能驅，此右病而左治之也。

Stomach Qi4 Pain

Patients, who fall sick and cannot take food and drink, have indigestion, stomach pain, stuffiness of stomach, or accompanied by vomiting diarrhea. These are all symptoms that liver wood restrains spleen earth. Formula:

白芍	bái sháo	Root of Paeonia lactiflora	2 qian
當歸	dāng guī	Root of Angelica polimorpha	2 qian
柴胡	chái hú	Root of Bupleurum chinense	2 qian
茯苓	fú líng	Dried fungus of Poria cocos	2 qian
白朮	bái zhú	Rhizome of Atractylodes macrocephala	3 qian
甘草	gān cǎo	Root of Glycyrrhiza uralensis	1 qian

白芥子	bái jiè zǐ	Seed of Brassica alba	1 qian

Two qian of **zhī zǐ** is added for fire and one qian of **ròu guì** for those without fire; Three qian of **shān zhā** added for food accumulation; One qian of **zhǐ ké** and two qian of **mài yá** are added for wheat-flour food damage; One qian of **bàn xià** is added for phlegm. Fire if there is any is dispersed and cold if any is dispelled. This is the right-sided disease treated from the left.

麻木門

Chapter 9 Numbness

手麻木

此乃氣虛而寒濕中之，如其不治，三年後必中大風，方用：

白朮、黃耆各伍錢，陳皮、桂枝各伍分，甘草壹兩，水煎服。

Hand Numbness and Insensitivity

Hand *numbness*[127] and insensitivity is the result of contraction of cold dampness during qi4 deficiency of patient. If not treated, patient will have violent wind stroke in three years. Formula:

白朮	bái zhú	Rhizome of Atractylodes macrocephala	5 qian
黃耆	huáng qí	Root of Astragalus membranaceus	5 qian
陳皮	chén pí	Peel of Citrus reticulata	5 fen
桂枝	guì zhī	Twigs of Cinnamonum cassia	5 fen
甘草	gān cǎo	Root of Glycyrrhiza uralensis	1 liang

127 *numbness*: reduced sensitivity to touch.

手麻

十指皆麻，面目失色，此亦氣虛也，治當補中益氣湯，加木香、麥冬、香附、羌活、烏藥、防風，三劑可愈。

Hand Numbness

Patient has ten numb fingers and lost his normal complexion as well as eye color. This is also qi4 deficiency. Proper therapy is the *Buzhong Yiqi Tang* [pinyin: bǔ zhōng yì qì tāng, 補中益氣湯, Central Qi4 Tonification Decoction] added with:

木香	mù xiāng	Root of Aucklandia lappa
麥冬	mài dōng	Tuber of Ophiopogon japonicus
香附	xiāng fù	Rhizome of Nutgrass Galingale
羌活	qiāng huó	Rhizome of Notopterygium forbesii Boiss.
烏藥	wū yào	Root of Combined Spicebush
防風	fáng fēng	Root of Ledebouriella divaricata

it cures in three doses.

手足麻木

手足麻木為中風之候，左右偏枯皆先由手足大指不用起，蓋手太陰肺經行於手大指，肺藏氣而右降，氣分虛則病偏於右，足厥陰肝經行於足大指，肝藏血而左升，血分虛則病偏於左，故手足麻木必補氣血，且驗中風之候於未來也。

四物湯加人參、白朮、茯苓、陳皮、半夏、桂枝、柴胡、羌活、防風、秦艽、牛膝炙草，薑、棗引煎服，四劑愈。

Numbness of Extremities

Numbness of extremities is a symptom of wind stroke. Either left or right hemiplegia begins with dysfunction of patient's thumb or toe, because the lung meridian (LU) moves through hand thumb, lung hoards qi4 and the right descends, qi4 aspect deficiency induces rightsided diseases; liver meridian (LR) moves through toe, liver hoards blood and the left ascends, qi4 aspect deficiency leads to leftsided diseases. Therefore, Qi4 and blood must be tonified for numbness of extremities, this also treats the symptoms of wind stroke before it strikes.

Si Wu Tang [pinyin: sì wù tāng, 四物湯, Four-medicinal Decoction] added with:

人參 rén shén Root of Panax ginseng

白术	bái zhú	Rhizome of Atractylodes macrocephala
茯苓	fú líng	Dried fungus of Poria cocos
陳皮	chén pí	Peel of Citrus reticulata
半夏	bàn xià	Rhizome of Pinellia ternata
桂枝	guì zhī	Twigs of Cinnamonum cassia
柴胡	chái hú	Root of Bupleurum chinense
羌活	qiāng huó	Rhizome of Notopterygium forbesii Boiss.
防風	fáng fēng	Root of Ledebouriella divaricata
秦艽	qín jiāo	Root of Gentiana macrophylla Pall.
牛膝	niú xī	Root of Achyranthes bidentata
灸草	jiǔ cǎo	Plant of Artemisia argyi

Accompanied by **jiāng** and **zǎo** as extra conductant ingredients, the formula cures numbness in four doses.

木

凡木是溼痰死血也，用四物湯加陳皮、半夏、茯苓、桃仁、紅花、白芥子、甘草、竹瀝、薑汁，水煎服。

Insensitivity

All insensitivity can be traced to damp phlegm and

dead blood. The prescription is *Siwu Tang* [pinyin: sì wù tāng, 四物湯, Four-medicinal Decoction] added with:

陳皮	chén pí	Peel of Citrus reticulata
半夏	bàn xià	Rhizome of Pinellia ternata
茯苓	fú líng	Dried fungus of Poria cocos
桃仁	táo rén	Seed of Prunus persica
紅花	hóng huā	Safflower
白芥子	bái jiè zǐ	Seed of Brassica alba
甘草	gān cǎo	Root of Glycyrrhiza uralensis
竹瀝	zhú lì	Sap of Phyllostachys
薑汁	jiāng zhī	Juice of common ginger

Preparation: Water decoction

腿麻木

方用導氣散：

黃耆貳錢、甘草壹錢伍分、青皮壹錢、升麻、柴胡、歸尾、澤瀉各伍分，五味子叁拾粒、陳皮捌分、紅花少許，水煎，溫服甚效。

Leg Numbness and Insensitivity

The prescription is Dao Qi San [pinyin: dǎo qì sǎn, 導氣散, Qi4-conducting Powder]:

黃耆	huáng qí	Root of Astragalus membranaceus	2 qian
甘草	gān cǎo	Root of Glycyrrhiza uralensis	1 qian 5 fen
青皮	qīng pí	Immature peel of Citrus reticulata	1 qian
升麻	shēng má	Rhizome of Cimifuga foetida	5 fen
柴胡	chái hú	Root of Bupleurum chinense	5 fen
歸尾	guī wěi	Prepared root of Radix Angelicae Sinensis	5 fen
澤瀉	zé xiè	Rhizome of Alisma plantago-aquatica	5 fen
五味子	wǔ wèi zǐ	Fruit of Schisandra chinensis	30 pieces
陳皮	chén pí	Peel of Citrus reticulata	8 fen
紅花	hóng huā	Safflower	a small amount

It is more effective to take the decoction warm.

兩手麻困倦嗜臥

此乃熱傷元氣也，方用益氣湯。

人參、甘草各壹錢、黃耆貳錢、炙草伍分、五味子參拾粒、柴胡、白芍各柒分、薑參片、棗貳枚，水煎熱服。

Numbness of Both Hands with Sleepiness and Somnolence

This is due to source qi4 hurt by heat, the prescription is *Yiqi Tang* [pinyin: yì qì tāng, 益氣湯, Qi4-tonifying Decoction]:

人參	rén shén	Root of Panax ginseng	1 qian
甘草	gān cǎo	Root of Glycyrrhiza uralensis	1 qian
黄耆	huáng qí	Root of Astragalus membranaceus	2 qian
炙草	jiǔ cǎo	Plant of Artemisia argyi	5 fen
五味子	wǔ wèi zǐ	Fruit of Schisandra chinensis	30 pieces
柴胡	chái hú	Root of Bupleurum chinense	7 fen
白芍	bái sháo	Root of Paeonia lactiflora	7 fen
薑	jiāng	Root of Zingiber officinale	3 slices
棗	zǎo	Fruit of Zizyphus jujuba	2 pieces

The water decoction shall be taken hot.

渾身麻木

凡人身體麻木不仁，兩目羞明怕日，眼澀難開，視物昏花，睛痛，方用神效黄耆湯。

黄耆、白芍各壹錢，陳皮伍分、人參捌分、炙草肆分、蔓荊子貳分。如有熱，加黃柏參分，水煎服。

Body Numbness and Insensitivity

The prescription is the *Shenxiao Huangqi Tang* [pinyin: shén xiào huáng qí tāng, 神效黃耆湯, Miraculously Efficacious Decoction of Root of Astragalus membranaceus] for symptoms of numb and insensitive body, that patient's eyes are afraid of brightness and sunshine and cannot open smoothly, dim eyesight and eye pain.

黃耆	huáng qí	Root of Astragalus membranaceus	1 qian
白芍	bái sháo	Root of Paeonia lactiflora	1 qian
陳皮	chén pí	Peel of Citrus reticulata	5 fen
人參	rén shēn	Root of Panax ginseng	8 fen
灸草	jiǔ cǎo	Plant of Artemisia argyi	4 fen
蔓荊子	màn jīng zǐ	Fruit of Simpleleaf shrub chastetree	2 fen

If there is fever, three fen of **huáng bǎi** is added.

麻木痛

風寒溼三氣，合而成疾，客於皮膚肌肉之間，或痛或麻木，方用：

牛膝膠貳兩、南星伍錢、薑汁半碗，共熬膏攤貼，再以熱鞋底熨之，加羌活、乳香、沒藥更妙。

Painful Numbness and Insensitivity

Wind, cold and dampness combine to form disease. Lingering in skin and muscles, they form pains, numbness and insensitivity. Formula:

牛膝胶 niú xī jiāo Jelly of root of Achyranthes bidentata 2 liang
南星 nán xīng Rhioze of Pinallianán xīng 5 qian
薑汁 jiāng zhī Juice of common ginger half bowelful

Medicinals are simmered together into ointment for application, then warm the area with hot sole of a shoe. It is better to add in **qiāng huó**, **rǔ xiāng**, and **mò yào**.

足弱

此症不能步履，人以為腎水之虛，誰知由於氣虛而不能運動乎，方用：

補中益氣湯加人參、牛膝各叁錢，金石斛伍錢、黃耆壹兩，水煎服。

Weak Feet

Patient with this symptom cannot walk. People think it is the deficiency of kidney water, though in fact inability in movement due to qi4 deficiency. The prescription is *Buzhong Yiqi Tang* [pinyin: bǔ zhōng yì qì tāng, 補中益氣湯, Central Qi Tonification Decoction] added with:

人參	rén shén	Root of Panax ginseng	3 qian
牛膝	niú xī	Root of Achyranthes bidentata	3 qian
金石斛	jīn shí hú	Whole plant of Dendrobii Nobilis	5 qian
黄耆	huáng qí	Root of Astragalus membranaceus	1 liang

筋縮

凡人一身筋脈，不可有病，病則筋縮而身痛，脈濇而體重矣，然筋之舒，在於血和，而脈之平，在於氣足，故治筋必須先治血，而治脈必須補氣，人若筋急拳縮傴僂，而不能直立者，皆筋病也，方用：

當歸壹兩、白芍、薏仁、生地、元參各伍錢，柴胡壹錢，水煎服。

此方妙在用柴胡一味，入於補藥中，蓋血虧則筋病，用補藥以治筋宜矣，何又用柴胡，夫肝為筋之主，筋乃肝之餘，氣不順，筋自縮急，今用柴胡以舒散之，鬱氣既除，而又濟之以大劑補血，則筋得其養矣。

Contracted Sinew

Sinews and vessels of human body shall not be sick, otherwise they *contract*[128] to cause pain of the body, rough pulse and heavy body. However, relaxation of sinews lies in harmonizing the blood and normality of vessels consists in sufficient qi4. Therefore, treatment of the sinews must begin with blood treatment, and treatment of the vessels must start from qi4 tonification. Patients' sinews huddle up to cause hunchback and they cannot rise to their feet, these are all symptoms of sinew disease. Formula:

當歸	dāng guī	Root of Angelica polimorpha	1 liang
白芍	bái sháo	Root of Paeonia lactiflora	5 qian
薏仁	yì rén	Seed kernel of Coix lachryma-jobi	5 qian

128 *contracted sinew*: permanent shortening of muscle with deformity and dysfunction.

生地 shēng dì Root of Rehmannia glutinosa Libosch. 5 qian

元参 yuán shēn Root of Scrophularia ningpoensis 5 qian

柴胡 chái hú Root of Bupleurum chinense 1 qian

The genius of this formula consists in its use of **chái hú** as a tonic. Blood deficiency gives rise to sinew diseases, so it is appropriate to employ tonics for treating sinews. Why is **chái hú** added? Liver is the principal of sinews and sinews are offshoots of the liver. If qi4 is not smooth, sinews will contract fast. Here, **chái hú** is employed to relax and dissipate, then stagnated qi4 is removed, after which large dose of blood-tonifying medicinals are applied so that sinews will be nourished.

脅痛門

Chapter 10 Costalgia

兩脅有塊

左脅有塊作痛，是死血也；右脅有塊作痛，是食積也。遍身作痛，筋骨尤甚，不能伸屈，口渴目赤，頭眩痰壅，胸不利，小便短赤，夜間殊甚，又遍身作痒如蟲行，人以為風也，誰知是腎氣虛而熱也。法用六味地黃湯加梔子、柴胡，是乃正治也。三劑見效。

Lumps on Both Sides of Chest

Painful lump on the left side of chest is of dead blood; Painful lump on the right side of chest is of food accumulation. Symptoms like pains all over the body, extremely painful sinews and bones that cannot extend or flex, thirst with red eyes and dizziness with phlegm blocked painful chest, oliguria with reddish urine that worsens during the night, body itches all over as if worms were crawling, are normally taken as wind. Who knows it is due to the heat of deficient kidney qi4? Proper therapy is *Liuwei Dihuang Tang* added with **zhī zǐ** and **chái hú**. This is an orthodox prescription, and efficacy will be sought in three three doses.

左脅痛

左脅痛，肝經受邪也。方用：

黃連吳萸炒貳錢，柴胡、當歸、青皮、桃仁研各壹錢，川芎捌分，紅花伍錢，水煎，食遠服。有痰，加陳皮、半夏。

Pain in the Left Side of Chest

Pain in the left side of chest is a symptom of pathogen-affected liver meridian. Formula:

黃連吳萸炒	huáng lián	Rhizome of Coptis chinensis (processed with Leaf of Trichotomous Evodia)	2 qian
柴胡	chái hú	Root of Bupleurum chinense	1 qian
當歸	dāng guī	Root of Angelica polimorpha	1 qian
青皮	qīng pí	Immature peel of Citrus reticulata	1 qian
桃仁	táo rén	Seed of Prunus persica (ground)	1 qian
川芎	chuān xiōng	Root of Ligusticum wallichii	8 fen
紅花	hóng huā	Safflower	5 qian

The water decoction shall be taken between meals. **Chén pí** and **bàn xià** are added for patients with phlegm.

右脅痛

此是邪入肺經也。方用：

片薑黃、枳殼各貳錢，桂心貳分，吳萸、陳皮、半夏各伍分，水煎服。

Pain in the Right Side of Chest

This is due to entrance of pathogens into the lung meridian. Formula:

片薑黃 piàn jiāng huáng Sliced flower of Hedychium coronarium Koenigt 2 qian

枳殼 zhǐ ké Dried peel of Aurantii fructus 2 qian

桂心 guì xīn Shaved inner bark of Cinnamonum cassia 2 fen

吳萸 wú yú Foliage of Trichotomous Evodia 5 fen

陳皮 chén pí Peel of Citrus reticulata 5 fen

半夏 bàn xià Rhizome of Pinellia ternata 5 fen

左右脅俱痛

方用：

柴胡、青皮、香附、龍膽草、當歸各一錢，川芎、枳殼各捌分，甘草參分，砂仁、木香各伍分，薑水煎服。

Pain in Both Sides of Chest

Formula:

柴胡	chái hú	Root of Bupleurum chinense	1 qian
青皮	qīng pí	Immature peel of Citrus reticulata	1 qian
香附	xiāng fù	Rhizome of Nutgrass Galingale	1 qian
龍膽草	lóng dǎn cǎo	Root and rhizome of Gentiana scabra	1 qian
當歸	dāng guī	Root of Angelica polimorpha	1 qian
川芎	chuān xiōng	Root of Ligusticum wallichii	8 fen
枳殼	zhǐ ké	Dried peel of Aurantii fructus	8 fen
甘草	gān cǎo	Root of Glycyrrhiza uralensis	3 fen
砂仁	shā rén	Fruit of Amomum villosum	5 fen
木香	mù xiāng	Root of Aucklandia lappa	5 fen

The medicinals are decocted with ginger.

兩脅走注

二陳湯去甘草，加枳殼、砂仁、廣木香、川芎、青皮、蒼朮、香附、茴香，水煎服。

Moving Pain in Both Sides of Chest

Moving pain in both sides of chest with patients' groan is due to phlegm. The prescription is *Ercheng Tang* [pinyin: èr chén tāng, 二陳湯, Two Old Medicinals Decoction]. **Gān cǎo** is deleted from the formula and added with:

砂仁	shā rén	Fruit of Amomum villosum
廣木香	mù xiāng	Root of Aucklandia lappa
川芎	chuān xiōng	Root of Ligusticum wallichii
青皮	qīng pí	Immature peel of Citrus reticulata
蒼朮	cāng zhú	Rhizome of Swordlike Atractylodes
香附	xiāng fù	Rhizome of Nutgrass Galingale
茴香	huí xiāng	Fruit of Foeniculum vulgare

脅痛身熱

此勞也。用補中益氣湯加川芎、白芍、青皮、砂仁、枳殼、茴香，去黃耆，水煎服。

Costalgia with Elevated Temperature

This is a consumptive disease. The prescription is *Buzhong Yiqi Tang* added with:

川芎	chuān xiōng	Root of Ligusticum wallichii
白芍	bái sháo	Root of Paeonia lactiflora
青皮	qīng pí	Immature peel of Citrus reticulata
砂仁	shā rén	Fruit of Amomum villosum
枳殼	zhǐ ké	Dried peel of Aurantii fructus
茴香	huí xiāng	Fruit of Foeniculum vulgare

But **huáng qí** shall be deleted from the original formula.

脅痛

此乃肝痛也。故治脅痛，必須平肝；平肝必須補腎；腎水足而後肝氣有養，不治脅痛，而脅痛自平也。方用肝腎兼資湯：

熟地、當歸各壹兩，白芍貳兩，黑梔壹錢，山萸伍錢，白芥子、甘草各叁錢，水煎服。

每咯血之人，脅漲痛而咯，是經血瘀滯脅下也，方用時加桃仁柒枚，黑荊芥穗捌分尤效。

Costalgia

Costalgia is a liver disease. To treat the costalgia, therefore, liver must be pacified which calls for the tonification of kidney. Sufficient kidney water brings about the nourished liver qi4. Costalgia will be gone though not treated directly. The prescription is *Ganshen Jianzi Tang* [pinyin: gān shèn jiān zī tāng, 肝腎兼資湯, Liver-kidney Dual Nourishment Decoction]

熟地 shú dì Prepared root of Rehmannia glutinosa 1 liang

當歸 dāng guī Root of Angelica polimorpha 1 liang

白芍 bái sháo Root of Paeonia lactiflora 2 liang

黑梔 hēi zhì Fruit or root of Gardenia stenphylla Merr. 1 qian

山萸 shān yú Fruit of Cornus officinalis 5 qian

白芥子 bái jiè zǐ Seed of Brassica alba 3 qian

甘草 gān cǎo Root of Glycyrrhiza uralensis 3 qian

Patients with hemoptysis often feel painful distension in both sides of chest and spit blood. This is meridian blood stagnated underneath his chest. Then seven pieces of **táo rén** and eight fen of **hēi jiè suì** shall be added to gain efficacy.

脅痛咳嗽

咳嗽氣急，脈滑數者，痰結痛也。

瓜蔞仁、枳殼、青皮、茴香、白芥子，水煎服。

Costalgia with Cough

Cough with shortness of breath and slippery and rapid pulse are symptoms of phlegm-binding pain.

瓜蔞仁	guā lóu rén	Seed of Trichosanthes kirilowii
枳殼	zhǐ ké	Dried peel of Aurantii fructus
青皮	qīng pí	Immature peel of Citrus reticulata
茴香	huí xiāng	Fruit of Foeniculum vulgare
白芥子	bái jiè zǐ	Seed of Brassica alba

濁淋門

Chapter 11

Turbid and Strangury Diseases

二濁五淋辨

濁淋二證，俱小便赤也。濁多虛，淋多實，淋痛、濁不痛為異耳。濁淋俱屬熱證，惟其不痛，大約屬溼痰下陷及脫精所致；惟其有痛，大約縱淫欲火動，強留敗精而然，不可混治。

Two Kinds of Turbid Diseases and Five Varieties of Strangury Diseases

Turbid and *strangury disease*[129] are both symptomized by reddish urine. The former is more of deficiency, and the latter is more of excess. Turbid disease has pains but strangury has not, this is the difference. They are both of heat diseases, but strangury has no pains. Strangury disease

129 *strangury disease*: a variety of diseases characterized by frequent, painful and dripping urination.

is due to sunken damp phlegm and *collapse of essence*[130], and turbid disease is due to overindulgence in sex that stirs fire, and forcible stoppage of ejaculation. These two diseases shall not be confused.

淋症

方用：五淋散。

淡竹葉、赤茯苓、芥穗、燈心各壹錢，車前子伍錢，水煎服。

Turbid Disease

Formula: *Wuling San* [pinyin: wǔ lín sǎn, 五淋散, Powder for Various Turbid Diseases]

淡竹葉	dàn zhú yè	Leaves of Lopatherum gracile	1 qian
赤茯苓	chì fú líng	Dried fungus of Rubra Poria	1 qian
芥穗	jiè suì	Spike of Fineleaf Schizonepeta	1 qian
燈心	dēng xīn	Pith of Junci Medulla	1 qian
車前子	chē qián zǐ	Seed of Plantago asiatica	5 qian

130 *collapse of essence*: a pathological change characterized by depletion and loss of kidney essence that leads to impaired hearing.

濁症

方用：清心蓮子飲。

石蓮子、人參各貳錢伍分，炙草、赤茯苓各貳錢，麥冬、黃耆、地骨皮、車前子各壹錢伍分，甘草伍分。水煎服。

Strangury Disease

Formula: *Qingxin Lianzi Yin* [pinyin: qīng xīn lián zǐ yǐn, 清心蓮子飲, Heart-clearing Lotus Seed Decoction]:

石蓮子 lián zǐ Seed of Nelumbo nucifera Gaerth 2 qian and 5 fen

人參 rén shén Root of Panax ginseng 2 qian and 5 fen

炙草 jiǔ cǎo Plant of Artemisia argyi 2 qian

赤茯苓 chì fú líng Dried fungus of Rubra Poria 2 qian

麥冬 mài dōng Tuber of Ophiopogon japonicus 1 qian and 5 fen

黃耆 huáng qí Root of Astragalus membranaceus 1 qian and 5 fen

地骨皮 dì gǔ pí Bark of the root of Lycium chinensis 1 qian and 5 fen

車前子 chē qián zǐ Seed of Plantago asiatica 1 qian and 5 fen

甘草 gān cǎo Root of Glycyrrhiza uralensis 5 fen

腎病門

Chapter 12 Kidney Diseases

陽強不倒

此虛火炎上，而肺氣不能下行故耳，若用黃柏知母煎湯飲之，立時消散，然自倒之後，終年不能振起，亦非善治之法也，方用：

元參、麥冬各參兩、肉桂參分，水煎服。

此方妙在用元參以瀉腎中之火，肉桂入其宅，麥冬助肺金之氣，清肅下行，以生腎水，水足則火自息矣，不求倒而自倒矣。

Priapism

This is due to upward flaming of deficiency fire and lung qi4's failure to descend. If treated with decoction of **huáng bǎi** and **zhī mǔ**, though the symptom disappears immediately upon intake of the decoction, patient will suffer from copulative impotency for a long time ever since.This is not a proper therapy. Formula:

元參 yuán shēn Root of Scrophularia ningpoensis 3 liang
麥冬 mài dōng Tuber of Ophiopogon japonicus 3 liang

肉桂 ròu guì   Bark of Cinnamonum cassia   3 fen

The genius of this formula consists in its use of **yuán shēn** that purges kidney fire. **Ròu guì** that enters its abode and **mài dōng** that assists with qi4 of lung metal. Clear qi4 descends to generate kidney water, and sufficient water means that fire will extinguish by itself. Symptom of priapism is gone even if not directly sought.

陽痿不舉

此症乃平日過於削，日泄其腎中之水，而腎中之火，亦因而消亡, 蓋水去而火亦去，必然之理，有如一家人口，廚下無水，何以為炊，必有水而後取柴炭以煮飯，不則空鐺也，方用：

熟地壹兩、山萸肆錢、遠志、巴戟、肉蓯蓉、杜仲各壹錢、肉桂、茯神各貳錢、白朮伍錢、人參叁錢，水煎服。

Impotence

This symptom is due to overindulgence in sex. Kidney water is ejaculated day by day and kidney fire disappears thereby since it is a universal truth that water retreats if fire is gone. This is comparable to family life. What to drink if there is no water in kitchen? Water is the first priority before firewood is sought for cooking. Otherwise, there are only empty cooking pots left. Formula:

熟地	shú dì	Prepared root of Rehmannia glutinosa	1 liang
山萸	shān yú	Fruit of Cornus officinalis	4 qian
遠志	yuǎn zhì	Root of Polygala tenuifolia	1 qian
巴戟	bā jǐ	Root of Morinda officinalis	1 qian
肉蓯蓉	ròu cōng róng	Fleshy stalk of Cistanche salsa	1 qian
杜仲	dù zhòng	Bark of Eucommia ulmoidis	1 qian
肉桂	ròu guì	Bark of Cinnamonum cassia	2 qian
茯神	fú shén	Sclerotium of Poria cocos	2 qian
白朮	bái zhú	Rhizome of Atractylodes macrocephala	5 qian
人參	rén shén	Root of Panax ginseng	3 qian

尿血又便血

便血出於後陰，尿血出於前陰，最難調治，然總之出血於下也，方用：

生地壹兩、地榆叁錢，水煎服，二症俱愈。蓋大小便各有經絡，而其症皆因膀胱之熱也，生地地榆，俱能清膀胱之熱，一方而兩用之也，蓋分之中有合。

Hematuria with Hematochezia

Bloody stool exits from *posterior yin*[131], and bloody urine discharges from the *anterior yin*[132]. These symptoms are the hardest to treat. But in general, it is bleeding from the under body. The formula:

生地 shēng dì Root of Rehmannia glutinosa Libosch.1 liang

地榆 dì yú Root of Sanguisorba officinalis 3 qian

Water decoction of the formula cures both symptoms. Excrement and urination are governed by own meridians and collaterals. The symptoms, nevertheless, are ascribable to heat of bladder which can be cleared away by **shēn dì** and **dì yú**. This is a dual application of one formula, since different symptoms have some points in common.

疝氣

方用去鈴丸：

大茴香、薑汁各壹斛，將薑汁入茴香內，侵一宿，入青鹽貳兩，同炒紅為末，酒丸桐子大，每服三十丸，溫酒或米湯送下。

[131] *posterior yin*: the anus, the posterior opening of the large intestine.

[132] *anterior yin:* the external genitalia including the external orifice of the urethra.

Genital Hernia

The formula is *Qu Ling Wan* [pinyin: qù ling wán, 去鈴丸, Bell-removing Pill]:

大茴香	dà huí xiāng	Fruit of Fructus Anisi Stellati	1 hu
薑汁	jiāng zhī	Juice of Common ginger	1 hu

Mix ginger juice with **huí xiāng** for extraction overnight, then add two liang of **qīng yán** and fry the mixture into red color and fine powder, then process into pills in size of tung-oil tree seed. Thirty pills are to be taken each time with lukewarm rice wine or thin rice gruel.

腎子痛

方用：

澤瀉、陳皮、赤苓各壹錢、丹皮、小茴香、枳實各叁錢、吳萸、蒼朮各伍分、山查肆分、蘇梗肆分，薑水煎服。又方：

酒炒大茴香、酒炒小茴香、赤石脂煅 、廣木香各等分，烏梅肉搗爛為丸，如桐子大，空心每服十五丸，蔥酒送下立效。

Testicle Pain

The formula:

澤瀉	zé xiè	Rhizome of Alisma plantago-aquatica	1 qian
陳皮	chén pí	Peel of Citrus reticulata	1 qian
赤苓	chì líng	Dried fungus of Rubra Poria	1 qian
丹皮	dān pí	Bark of the root of Paeonia suffruticosa	3 qian
小茴香	xiǎo huí xiāng	Fruit of Foeniculum vulgare	3 qian
枳實	zhǐ shí	Unripe fruit of Poncirus trifoliate	3 qian
吳萸	wú yú	Leaf of Trichotomous Evodia	5 fen
蒼朮	cāng zhú	Rhizome of Swordlike Atractylodes	5 fen
山查	shān zhā	Fruit of Crateagus pinnatifida	4 fen
蘇梗	sū gěng	Herb of Perilla frutescens L. Britt.	4 fen

Ginger water decoction. Another formula:

To process equal amount of **dà huí xiāng** wine processed, **xiǎo huí xiāng** wine processed, **chì shí zhī** calcined, **guǎng mù xiāng** and pulp of **wū méi ròu** into pills in size of tung-oil tree seed. Fifteen pills are to be taken each time with green onion wine when stomach is empty. The efficacy is instantaneous.

偏墜

方用：

小茴香、豬苓等分，微炒為末，空心鹽水沖服，熱鹽熨亦甚效。

Unilateral Swollen Testicle

The formula:

Equal weight of **xiǎo huí xiāng** and **zhū ling** are slightly fried and processed into fine powder which is to be *taken drenched*[133] with salt solution when stomach is empty. *Hot medicinal compress*[134] with salt is very effective as well.

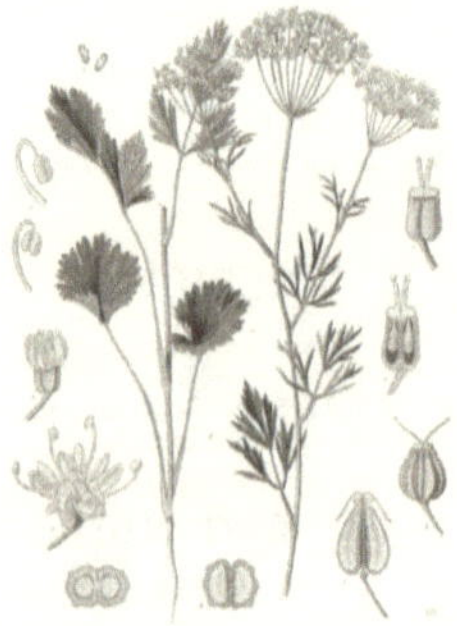

[133] *take drenched*: take medicine after pouring hot water or hot decoction of other medicinals over it, with stirring.

[134] *hot medicinal compress*: a therapeutic measure involving pressing and rubbing the diseased area with hot medical substances wrapped in cloth.

雜 方

Chapter 13 Miscellaneous Formulae

病在上而求諸下

頭痛、目痛、耳紅、腮腫，一切上焦等症，除清涼發散正治外，人即束手無策，而不知更有三法。

如大便結、脈沉實者，用酒蒸大黃三錢微下之，名釜底抽薪之法；如大便瀉，脈沉足冷者，宜六味地黃湯，加牛膝、車前、肉桂，足冷甚者，加熟附子，是冷極於下，而迫其火之上升也，此名導龍入海之法；大便如常，脈無力者，用牛膝車前引下之，此名引火歸源之法也。

To Seek Treatment of Upper Diseases from the Lower

All symptoms of upper energizer such as headache, eye pain, reddened ears, and mumps are treated with orthodox medicinals of cool and dispersing property, aside from which, practitioners are rather helpless and ignorant of the following three therapies.

For patients with symptoms of hard bound stool and replete and heavy pulse, three qian of **dà huáng** steamed in wine is used for a slight purgation, which is knows as the therapy of "removing the burning wood from under the boiler" ; For those with symptoms of diarrhea, heavy pulse and cold feet, *Liuwei Dihuang Tang* with addition of **niú xī**, **chē qian** and **ròu guì** is a proper prescription. For patients with utmost foot coldness, **shú fù zǐ** is added. The extreme lower coldness forces fire to flame upwards. This therapy is named as "Conducting Dragon into Ocean"; For those with normal stool but weak pulse, **niú xī** and **chē qián** are employed to *conduct fire back to its origin*[135].

病在下而求諸上

凡治下焦病用本藥不愈者，須從上治之。

如足痛足腫，無力虛軟，膝瘡紅腫，用木瓜、薏仁、牛膝、防已、黃柏、蒼朮之品，不效者定是中氣下陷，溼熱下流，用補中益氣升提之；

如足軟不能行而能食，名曰痿症，宜清肺熱；

如治泄瀉，用實脾利水之劑，不效者亦用補中益氣，

---

[135] *conduct fire back to its origin*: a therapeutic principle for the ascending of asthenic fire, by adding drugs for tonifying the kidney yang to those for nourishing the kidney yin to lead the ascending deficiency fire back down to the kidney, the same as to conduct fire downward.

去當歸，加炮薑、蒼朮，脈遲加肉蔻、故紙；

如尿血、用涼血利水藥不效，宜清心蓮子飲，若清心不止，再加升柴；

如治便血，用止濯之藥，不效或兼泄瀉，須察其脈，如右關微或數大無力，是脾虛不攝血，宜六君子加炮薑，若右關沉緊，是飲食傷脾，不能攝血，加沉香貳分，右寸洪數，是實熱在肺，宜清肺，麥冬、花粉、元參、枯芩、桔梗、五味子、枳殼等味。

To Seek Treatment of Lower Body Diseases from the Upper

The diseases of lower energizer incurable with orthodox medicinals shall be treated from the upper.

As for symptoms of foot pain, swollen feet, weakness, and reddish swollen knee sore, they shall be treated with medicinals like **mù guā**, **yì rén**, **niú xī**, **fáng jǐ**, **huáng bǎi**, **cāng zhú** and so on. If not effective, it is certainly due to sunken middle qi4 and downward-flowing of damp heat, which should be remedied by *Bu Zhong Yi qi Tang* for upraising.

Patients capable of food intake but unable to walk for their soft feet must have wilting diseases and shall be treated by clearing lung heat.

Patients with diarrhea shall be treated with medicinals that fortify spleen and induce diuresis. If not effective, *Bu Zhong Yi qi Tang* should be employed though without **dāng guī** and added with **pào jiāng** and **cāng zhú**. **Ròu kòu** and **gù zhǐ** are added for those with slow pulse.

For patients with hematuria and incurable if treated with blood-cooling and diuresis-inducing medicinals, *Qingxin Lianzi Yin* is to be prescribed. If pathogens are not cleared away from the pericardium, **shēng má** and **chái hú** shall be added.

Patients with hematochezia shall be treated with astringency-relieving medicinals. If ineffective or patient is complicated with diarrhea, his pulse must be taken. If the right guan is faint, or rapid and large, this is a sign of deficient spleen unable to control blood and should be treated with *Liujunzi Tang* added with **pào jiāng**. If the right guan is heavy and tight, it is a sign of spleen damaged by food intake and unable to control blood, two fen of **chén xiāng** is added. If the right cun is surging and rapid, this is excessive heat in lung, and should be treated with lung-clearing medicinals like **mài dōng**, **huā fěn**, **yuán shēn**, **kū qín**, **jié gěng**, **wǔ wèi zǐ**, **zhǐ ké**, etc.

瘡毒

方用如神湯:

銀花、當歸、蒲公英各壹兩、荊芥、連翹各壹錢、甘草叁錢，水煎服。

Poisoned Sore

The formula is *Rushen Tang* [pinyin: rú shén tāng, 如神湯, Para Miraculous Decoction]:

銀花	yín huā	Flower of Lonicera japonica	1 liang
當歸	dāng guī	Root of Angelica polimorpha	1 liang
蒲公英	pú gōng yīng	Herb of Herba Taraxaci	1 liang
荊芥	jīng jiè	Leaf of Schizonepeta tenuifolia	1 qian
連翹	lián qiào	Fruit of Forsythia suspensa(Thunb.)Vahl	1 qian
甘草	gān cǎo	Root of Glycyrrhiza uralensis	3 qian

頭面上瘡

方用：

銀花貳兩、當歸壹兩、川芎、甘草各伍錢、桔梗、蒲公英各叁錢、黃芩壹錢，水煎服，二劑全消。

頭瘡不可用升提之藥，最宜用降火之品，切記之。

Sore on Head and Face

Formula:

銀花	yín huā	Flower of Lonicera japonica	2 liang
當歸	dāng guī	Root of Angelica polimorpha	1 liang
川芎	chuān xiōng	Root of Ligusticum wallichii	5 qian
甘草	gān cǎo	Root of Glycyrrhiza uralensis	5 qian
桔梗	jié gěng	Root of Platycodon grandiflorum	3 qian
蒲公英	pú gōng yīng	Herb of Herba Taraxaci	3 qian
黃芩	huáng qín	Root of Scutellaria baicalensis	1 qian

Water decoction, it cures in two doses. Sores on head shall not be treated with upraising medicinals, but it is appropriate to use fire down-bearing ones. This point must be remembered clearly.

身上手足之瘡疽

方用：

銀花、甘草、蒲公英各叁錢、當歸壹兩、牛蒡子貳錢、花粉伍錢、芙蓉葉七片，無葉用根，水煎服。

Scabies on Body and Extremities

Formula:

銀花	yín huā	Flower of Lonicera japonica	3 qian
甘草	gān cǎo	Root of Glycyrrhiza uralensis	3 qian
蒲公英	pú gōng yīng	Herb of Herba Taraxaci	3 qian
當歸	dāng guī	Root of Angelica polimorpha	1 liang
牛蒡子	niú bàng zǐ	Root of Arctium lappa	2 qian
花粉	huā fěn	Seed of Trichosanthes kirilowii	5 qian
芙蓉葉	fú róng yè	Foliage of Coffonrose Hibiscus	7 pieces

(if without, root is also applicable)

統治諸瘡

方用：

花粉、甘草、銀花、蒲公英， 水煎服，二劑全愈。此方消毒大有其功，諸癰諸疽，不論部位，皆治之。

For All Kinds of Sores

Formula:

花粉	huā fěn	Seed of Trichosanthes kirilowii
甘草	gān cǎo	Root of Glycyrrhiza uralensis
銀花	yín huā	Flower of Lonicera japonica

蒲公英 pú gōng yīng Herb of Herba Taraxaci

It cures in two doses. This formula is extremely effective for detoxification, and can be applied in treating any kinds of abscesses and sores on whatever part of human body.

黄水瘡

方用：

雄黄、防風煎湯，洗之即愈。

Yellow Water Sore

Formula:

The sore cures to wash with the decoction of **xióng huáng** and **fáng fēng**.

手汗

方用：

黄耆、乾葛各壹兩、荊芥、防風各叁錢，水煎壹盆，熱薰溫洗，三次愈。

Hand Perspiration

Formula:

黄耆 huáng qí Root of Astragalus membranaceus 1 liang

乾葛	gān gé	Root of Pueraria lobata	1 liang
荊芥	jīng jiè	Leaf of Schizonepeta tenuifolia	3 qian
防風	fáng fēng	Root of Ledebouriella divaricata	3 qian

One basin of water decoction for hot fumigation and warm wash, it cures in three doses.

飲砒毒

用生甘草參兩，加羊血半碗，和勻飲之，立吐而愈，若不吐，速用大黃貳兩、甘草伍錢，白礬壹兩，當歸參兩，水煎數碗飲之，立時大瀉即生。

Intoxication of White Arsenic

Mix up well two liang of **shēng gān cǎo** and a half bowl of sheep blood and drink immediately. It cures if patient vomits. Otherwise, instantly decoct two liang **dà huáng** and five qian of **gān cǎo**, one liang of **bái fán** and three liang of **dāng guī** into a few bowls of decoction for intake. Patient will be saved if he has a big loose bowl after taking the decoction.

補腎

方用：

大鹽青菽葦七寸，煮核桃。

Kidney Tonification

The formula:

To decocted seven *cun*[136] of green soybean leaves and a large amount of Salt (sodium chloride) together with **hé tao**.

嚏噴

方用：

生半夏為末，水丸綠豆大，入鼻孔，必嚏噴不已，用水飲之立止，通治中風不語，及中惡中鬼俱妙。

Sneeze

Formula:

Grind **shēng bàn xià** into powder so as to prepare water pills in size of mung bean. Apply into nostrils, the patient cannot help but sneeze, let patient take water and the sneeze is gone at once. The formula is also applicable to wind stroke with aphasia and pestilent or evil factor attack.

---

136 *cun:* A length unit of ancient China, 1 cun equals 3.33 cm.

破傷风

方用：

蟬退去淨頭足為末伍錢，用好酒壹碗，煎滚入末，調匀服之，立生。

Tetanus

The formula:

Grind **chán tuì** without head and legs into five qian of fine powder, boil one bowl of good wine to mix up with the powder for intake. Patient survives then.

瘋狗咬傷

用：

手指甲焙黄為末，滚黄酒沖服，發汗即愈，忌房事百日。

Bite by Mad Dog

Therapy:

Fingernail baked into yellow color and ground to powder, take drenched with boiling rice wine and it cures after patient's sweating. Sexual activity should be prohibited for a hundred days.

小兒科

Chapter 14 Pediatrics

色

小兒鼻之上、眼之中色紅者，心熱也；紅筋橫直，現於山根，皆心熱也；色紫者，心熱之甚而肺亦熱也；色青者，肝有風也；青筋橫直現者，肝熱也，直者，風上行；橫者風下行也；色黑者，風甚而腎中有寒也；色白者，肺中有痰；黃者脾胃虛而作瀉。一觀其色，而疾可知矣。

Color

Red color in children's eyes and on their noses is heart heat, and the appearance of crisscrossed reddish veins on the *root of nose*[137] is heart heat too. Purple color stands for utmost heart heat accompanied by lung heat; Bluish color stands for liver wind; Bluish veins crisscrossed is liver heat, and vertical veins is a symptom of upraising wind while horizontal veins is a symptom of descending wind; Dark

[137] *root of nose*: the upper portion of the nose, which is situated between the eyes, the same as radix nasi.

color means the wind is utmost and there is cold in kidney; White color means there is phlegm in lung while yellow color means that spleen-stomach is deficient and there is a tendency to diarrhea. Diseases are diagnosed once the color is observed.

脈

大人看脈於寸、關、尺，小兒不然，但看其數不數而已。數甚則熱，不數則寒也；數之中浮者，風也；沉者，寒也；緩者，溼也；濇者，邪也；滑者，痰也；有止歇者，痛也；如此而已，餘不必過談也。

Pulse

An adult's pulse is taken at *cun, guan and chi*[138], but it is a different case for children. We only need to take whether it is rapid or not. Rapid pulse is a heat and non-rapid pulse is a cold one. Rapid pulse with floating is wind; it is cold if

138 *cun, guan and chi:* the 3 sections over the radial artery for feeling the pulse: The bar/guan is just central to the radial styloid at the wrist, where the tip of the physician's middle finger is placed, the inch/cun is next to it on the distal side where the tip of the physician's index finger rests, and the cubit/chi is on the proximal side where the tip of the physician's ring finger is placed.

with *sunken pulse*[139]; it is dampness if with *relaxed pulse*[140]; it is pathogen if with *rough pulse*[141]; it is phlegm if with slippery pulse and it is pain if with pauses. This is all, and there is no necessity to make further ado.

三關

小兒虎口，風氣命三關，紫屬熱，紅屬寒，青屬驚風，白屬疳，風關輕，氣為重，若至命關，則難治矣。

Three Bars

Wind bar, qi4 bar and life bar are known as the tiger-mouth *three bars*[142] of children. Purple color belongs to heat; red color belongs to cold; bluish color belongs to *infantile convulsion*[143]; And white color belongs to *infantile*

---

[139] *sunken pulse:* a deeply located pulse which can only be felt when pressing hard, also called deep pulse.

[140] *relaxed pulse*: a pulse with decreased tension. It is different from another 緩脈 (Pinyin: huǎn mài) which means moderate pulse, a pulse with 4 beats to 1 cycle of the physician's respiration, even and harmonious in its form.

[141] *rough pulse:* a pulse coming and going unsmoothly with small, fine, slow joggling tempo like scraping bamboo with a knife.

[142] *Three bars:* a collective term for the 3 segments of the index finger used for measuring the extension of the visible venules, i.e., "wind bar", "qi4 bar" and "life bar", also known as 3 gates.

[143] *infantile convulsion:* infantile diseases marked by convulsions and

malnutrition; If the wind bar is light, the qi4 is heavy and if developinged to the life bar, it is hard to treat.

不食乳

小兒不食乳，心熱也，蔥煎乳汁，令小兒服之亦妙，不若用黃連三分，煎湯一分，灌數次即食矣，神效。

Milk Apastia

That children refuse to take milk is a symptom of heart heat. It is good to let children take milk decocted with green onion, but it is better to have three fen of **huáng lián** decocted. Patient starts to take food after taking the decoction several times, and it is miraculously effective.

臍不乾

用車前子炒焦為細末，敷之即乾。

Umbilical Dampness

Formula for *umbilical dampness*[144]:

---

loss of consciousness.

144 *umbilical dampness*: a condition of wetness of and possible exudation from the umbilicus after the umbilical cord has been shed, referring to

Parch **chē qián zǐ** into brown and grind the medicinal into fine powder, it dries after applying the powder to the navel part.

山根

山根之上，有青筋直現者，乃肝熱也。方用：

柴胡、半夏各參分，白芍、茯苓各壹錢，當歸、白朮各伍分，山查參箇，甘草壹分，水煎服。

有青筋橫現者，亦肝熱也。直者風上行，橫者風下行。用前方加柴胡伍分，麥芽壹錢，乾薑壹分，水煎服。

有紅筋直現者，心熱也。亦用前方加黃連壹分，麥冬伍分，去半夏，加桑白皮、天花粉各貳分，水煎服。

有紅筋斜現者，亦心熱也。亦用前方加黃連貳分，熱積於胸中，不可用半夏，用桑白皮、花粉可也。

有黃筋現於山根者，不論橫直，總是脾胃之證，或吐或瀉，腹痛或不思食。方用：

白朮、茯苓各伍分，陳皮、人參、麥芽各貳分，神麯、甘草各壹分，淡竹葉柒分，水煎服。

有痰加半夏壹分，白芥子貳分；如口渴有熱者，加麥冬參分，黃芩壹分；有寒加乾薑壹分；吐加白蔻壹粒；瀉

---

omphalorrhea.

加豬苓伍分；腹痛按之大叫者，食也，加大黃參分，枳實壹分；按之不呼號者，寒也，加乾薑參分；如身發熱者，不可用此方。

The Root of Nose

That bluish veins are obviously visible on the root of nose is a sign of liver heat. Formula:

柴胡	chái hú	Root of Bupleurum chinense	3 fen
半夏	bàn xià	Rhizome of Pinellia ternata	3 fen
白芍	bái sháo	Root of Paeonia lactiflora	1 qian
茯苓	fú líng	Dried fungus of Poria cocos	1 qian
當歸	dāng guī	Root of Angelica polimorpha	5 fen
白术	bái zhú	Rhizome of Atractylodes macrocephala	5 fen
山查	shān zhā	Fruit of Crateagus pinnatifida	3 pieces
甘草	gān cǎo	Root of Glycyrrhiza uralensis	1 fen

That bluish veins are horizontal in order is also a symptom of liver heat. For vertical cases the wind goes upward, and for horizontal cases the wind goes down. The prescription is the former formula added with:

柴胡	chái hú	Root of Bupleurum chinense	5 fen
麥芽	mài yá	Sprout of Oryza sativa	1 qian
乾薑	gān jiāng	Dried Common ginger	1 fen

That reddish veins in vertical order are also a sign of heart fire. The prescription is the former formula added with:

黃連	huáng lián	Rhizome of Coptis chinensis	1 fen
麥冬	mài dōng	Tuber of Ophiopogon japonicus	5 fen
桑白皮	sāng bái pí	Bark of the root of Morus alba	2 fen
天花粉	tiān huā fěn	Seed of Trichosanthes kirilowii	2 fen

Bàn xià shall be deleted from the formula.

That the reddish veins shown in an oblique way are as well a symptom of heart fire. We also use the forma formula added with two fen of **huáng lián**. Since heat accumulates in chest, we cannot use **bàn xià**, but **sāng bái pí** and **tiān huā fěn**.

That yellowish veins shown on the root of nose, whether in horizontal or vertical order, are invariably a sign of spleen-stomach disease. Patients either vomit or have diarrhea, stomachache or poor appetite. Formula:

白术	bái zhú	Rhizome of Atractylodes macrocephala	5 fen
茯苓	fú líng	Dried fungus of Poria cocos	5 fen
陳皮	chén pí	Peel of Citrus reticulata	2 fen
人參	rén shén	Root of Panax ginseng	2 fen
麥芽	mài yá	Sprout of Oryza sativa	2 fen
神麴	shén qū	Medicated leaven	1 fen
甘草	gān cǎo	Root of Glycyrrhiza uralensis	1 fen
淡竹葉	dàn zhú yè	Leaves of Lopatherum gracile	7 fen

If patients have phlegm, one fen of **bàn xià** and two fen of **bái jiè zi3** are added. If they are thirsty, three fen of **mài dōng** and one fen of **huáng qín** are added. If they have cold, one fen of **gān jiāng** is added. If they vomit, one piece of **bái kòu** is added. If they have diarrhea, five fen of **zhū ling** are added. If patient has abdomen pains and yells once pressed, this is food damage and shall be treated with three fen of **dà huáng**, one fen of **zhǐ shí**. If patient does not yell once pressed, this is cold, three fen of **gān jiāng** should be added. This formula is not applicable to those with elevated temperature.

發熱

不拘早晚發熱，俱用萬全湯，神效。

柴胡、白朮、黃芩、神麴各參分，白芍、麥冬各壹錢，當歸伍分，茯苓三分，甘草、蘇葉各壹分，山查參箇，水煎服。

冬加麻黃壹分，夏加石膏參分，春加青蒿參分，秋加桔梗參分，有食加枳殼參分，有痰加白芥子參分，吐加白蔻壹粒，瀉加豬苓壹錢。小兒諸證，不過如此，不可作驚風治之。如果有驚風，加人參伍分，其效如神。

凡潮熱、積熱、瘧熱，乃脾積寒熱，俱用薑梨引。

柴胡、人參、黃芩、前胡、秦艽、甘草、青蒿各壹分，童便浸曬乾，生地一寸，薄荷二葉，或生梨、生藕一片，水煎服，甚效。

Fever

Whether for morning fever or night fever, *Wanquan Tang* [pinyin: wàn quán tāng, 萬全湯, Safe and Sound Decoction] is miraculously effective:

柴胡	chái hú	Root of Bupleurum chinense	3 fen
白朮	bái zhú	Rhizome of Atractylodes macrocephala	3 fen

黄芩	huáng qín	Root of Scutellaria baicalensis	3 fen
神麴	shén qū	Medicated leaven	3 fen
白芍	bái sháo	Root of Paeonia lactiflora	1 qian
麥冬	mài dōng	Tuber of Ophiopogon japonicus	1 qian
當歸	dāng guī	Root of Angelica polimorpha	5 fen
茯苓	fú líng	Dried fungus of Poria cocos	2 fen
甘草	gān cǎo	Root of Glycyrrhiza uralensis	1 fen
蘇葉	sū yè	Foliage of Perilla frutescens	1 fen
山查	shān zhā	Fruit of Crateagus pinnatifida	3 pieces

One fen of **má huáng** is added in winter, three fen of **shí gāo** is added in summer; Three fen of **qīng hāo** is added in spring, and three fen of **jié gěng** is added in autumn. Three fen of **zhǐ ké** is added for food damage, three fen of **bái jiè zi3** is added for phlegm, one piece of **bái kòu** is added for vomit, and one qian of **zhū ling** is added for diarrhea. The medicaments for children's diseases are just like this, they should not be treated as infantile convulsion. If with infantile convulsion, addition of five fen of **rén shén** is miraculously effective.

Tidal fever, accumulated heat, malaria heat are all due

to accumulated cold or heat at spleen, and should be treated with *Jiangli Yin* [pinyin: jiāng lí yǐn, 薑梨引, Ginger and Pear Decoction]:

Immerse one fen of **chái hú**, **rén shén**, **huáng qín**, **qián hú**, **qín jiāo**, **gān cǎo**, and **qīng hāo** respectively in boy's urine and dry up, then decoct the medicinals with one cun of **shēng dì** and two pieces of **bò he** or a piece of raw pear or raw lotus root. The decoction is truly effective.

感冒風寒

方用：

柴胡伍分，白朮、白芍各壹錢，茯苓、炙草、半夏各參分，陳皮貳分，當歸捌分，水煎熱服。

Common Cold and Wind-cold

Formula:

柴胡	chái hú	Root of Bupleurum chinense	5 fen
白术	bái zhú	Rhizome of Atractylodes macrocephala	1 qian
白芍	bái sháo	Root of Paeonia lactiflora	1 qian
茯苓	fú líng	Dried fungus of Poria cocos	3 fen
炙草	jiǔ cǎo	Plant of Artemisia argyi	3 fen

半夏	bàn xià	Rhizome of Pinellia ternata	3 fen
陳皮	chén pí	Peel of Citrus reticulata	2 fen
當歸	dāng guī	Root of Angelica polimorpha	8 fen

Decoction should be taken hot.

驚風

世人動曰驚風，誰知小兒驚則有之，而風則無。小兒純陽之體，不當有風，而狀有風者，蓋小兒陽旺內熱，內熱則生風，是非外來之風，乃內出之風也。內風作外風治，是速之死也，方用清火散風湯：

白朮、梔子各參分，茯苓貳錢，陳皮、甘草、半夏各壹分，白芍壹錢，柴胡伍分，水煎服。

此方健脾平肝之聖藥，肝平則火散，脾健則風止，斷不可以風藥表散之也。

Infantile Convulsion

People often name it "wind fright" instead of infantile convulsion, though in fact there are frights, but there is no wind. Child has a pure yang body and can hardly be affected by wind. Those seemingly wind symptoms are in fact internal heat of yang excess of them. Internal heat leads to wind, a wind from the interior of body instead of the exterior. If treated as external wind, the child may soon die. The prescription is *Qinghuo Sanfeng Tang* [qīng huǒ sàn fēng tāng, 清火散風湯, Fire-clearing and Wind-dispersing Decoction]:

白术	bái zhú	Rhizome of Atractylodes macrocephala	3 fen
梔子	zhī zǐ	Fruit of Gardenia jasminoides	3 fen
茯苓	fú líng	Dried fungus of Poria cocos	2 qian
陳皮	chén pí	Peel of Citrus reticulata	1 fen
甘草	gān cǎo	Root of Glycyrrhiza uralensis	1 fen
半夏	bàn xià	Rhizome of Pinellia ternata	1 fen
白芍	bái sháo	Root of Paeonia lactiflora	1 qian
柴胡	chái hú	Root of Bupleurum chinense	5 fen

This is a sovereign remedy for spleen fortification and liver pacification. The fire goes since liver is pacified, and the wind stops since spleen is fortified. The wind should never be treated with exterior-dissipating medicinal

驚風

凡驚風皆由於氣虛，方用壓風湯：

人參、白朮、神麴各伍分，甘草、半夏、丹砂各參分，茯神壹錢，砂仁壹粒，陳皮壹分，水煎服。

此方治慢驚風，加黃耆。

Infantile Convulsion

All infantile convulsion originates from qi4 deficiency, The prescription is *Yafeng Tang* [pinyin: yā fēng tāng, 壓風湯, Wind-controlling Decoction]:

人參	rén shén	Root of Panax ginseng	5 fen
白朮	bái zhú	Rhizome of Atractylodes macrocephala	5 fen
神麴	shén qū	Medicated leaven	5 fen
甘草	gān cǎo	Root of Glycyrrhiza uralensis	3 fen
半夏	bàn xià	Rhizome of Pinellia ternata	3 fen
丹砂	dān shā	Mercuric sulfide	3 fen
茯神	fú shén	Sclerotium of Poria cocos	1 qian
砂仁	shā rén	Fruit of Amomum villosum	1 piece
陳皮	chén pí	Peel of Citrus reticulata	1 fen

For chronic infantile convulsion, **huáng qí** shall be added.

痢疾

方用：

當歸、白芍各壹錢，黃連貳分，枳殼、檳榔各伍分，甘草參分，水煎溫服。

紅痢倍黃連，白痢加澤瀉參分，腹痛倍甘草加白芍，小便赤加木通參分，下如豆汁，加白朮壹錢，傷食加山查、麥芽各參分，氣虛加人參參分。

Dysentery

Formula:

當歸	dāng guī	Root of Angelica polimorpha	1 qian
白芍	bái sháo	Root of Paeonia lactiflora	1 qian
黃連	huáng lián	Rhizome of Coptis chinensis	2 fen
枳殼	zhǐ ké	Dried peel of Aurantii fructus	5 fen
檳榔	bīng láng	Fruit of Areca catechu	5 fen
甘草	gān cǎo	Root of Glycyrrhiza uralensis	3 fen

Decoction should be taken warm.

For red dysentery, two times of **huáng lián** is used, and for white dysentery three fen of **zé xiè** is added; For painful abdomen, two times of **gān cǎo** is used together with **bái sháo**; For reddish urine, three fen of **mù tōng** is added. For milk-like urine, one qian of **bái zhú** is added; For food damage, three fen of **shān zhā** and three fen of **mài yá** are added; For qi4 deficiency, three fen of **rén shén** is added.

泄瀉

身熱如火，口渴舌燥，喜冷飲而不喜熱湯。方用瀉火止瀉湯：

車前子貳錢，茯苓、白芍、麥芽各壹錢，黃連、豬苓各參分，澤瀉伍分，枳殼貳分，水煎服。

Diarrhea

Patient's body is as hot as fire, he is thirst and his tongue is dry. He prefers cold drinks instead of hot water. The formula is *Xiehuo Zhixie Tang* [pinyin: xiè huǒ zhǐ xiè tāng, 瀉火止瀉湯, Fire-purging and Diarrhea-stopping Decoction]:

車前子	chē qián zǐ	Seed of Plantago asiatica	2 qian
茯苓	fú líng	Dried fungus of Poria cocos	1 qian
白芍	bái sháo	Root of Paeonia lactiflora	1 qian
麥芽	mài yá	Sprout of Oryza sativa	1 qian
黃連	huáng lián	Rhizome of Coptis chinensis	3 fen
豬苓	zhū líng	Agaric Polyporus	3 fen
澤瀉	zé xiè	Rhizome of Alisma plantago-aquatica	5 fen
枳殼	zhǐ ké	Dried peel of Aurantii fructus	2 fen

寒瀉

此症必腹痛而喜手按摩，口不渴而舌滑，喜熱飲而不喜冷水也。方用散寒止瀉湯：

人參、白朮各壹錢，茯苓貳錢，肉桂、乾薑各貳分，甘草壹分，砂仁壹粒，神麴伍分，水煎服。

Cold Diarrhea

Cold diarrhea must have symptoms of abdominal pain that may relieve if massaged, slippery tongue without thirst, and patient likes hot drinks instead of cold. The formula is *Sanhan Zhixie Tang* [pinyin: sàn hán zhǐ xiè tāng, **散寒止瀉**

湯, Decoction for Dispelling coldness and Stopping diarrhea]:

人參	rén shēn	Root of Panax ginseng	1 qian
白术	bái zhú	Rhizome of Atractylodes macrocephala	1 qian
茯苓	fú líng	Dried fungus of Poria cocos	2 qian
肉桂	ròu guì	Bark of Cinnamomum cassia	2 fen
幹薑	gān jiāng	Dried Common ginger	2 fen
甘草	gān cǎo	Root of Glycyrrhiza uralensis	1 fen
砂仁	shā rén	Fruit of Amomum villosum	1 piece
神麴	shén qū	Medicated leaven	5 fen

吐

此證雖胃氣之弱，亦脾氣之虛。小兒恣意飽食，不能消化，久之上沖於胃口而吐也，方用止吐速效湯：

人參、白朮各壹錢，砂仁壹粒，茯苓貳錢，陳皮貳分，麥芽伍分，半夏、乾薑各壹分，山查參箇，水煎服。

Vomit

This symptom is due to weakness of stomach qi4 as well as deficiency of spleen qi4. Children are willful in food intake though they cannot digest properly, which in a long run, will rush upward to the mouth of stomach to form vomit. The prescription is *Zhitu Suxiao Tang* [pinyin: zhǐ tù sù xiào tāng, 止吐速效湯, Vomit-stopping Decoction of Quick Result]:

人參	rén shén	Root of Panax ginseng	1 qian
白术	bái zhú	Rhizome of Atractylodes macrocephala	1 qian
砂仁	shā rén	Fruit of Amomum villosum	1 piece
茯苓	fú líng	Dried fungus of Poria cocos	2 qian
陳皮	chén pí	Peel of Citrus reticulata	2 fen
麥芽	mài yá	Sprout of Oryza sativa	5 fen
半夏	bàn xià	Rhizome of Pinellia ternata	1 fen
乾薑	gān jiāng	Dried Common ginger	1 fen
山查	shān zhā	Fruit of Crateagus pinnatifida	3 pieces

咳嗽

方用：

蘇葉伍分，桔梗、甘草各壹錢，水煎熱服。有痰加白芥子伍分便是。

Cough

Formula:

蘇葉	sū yè	Foliage of Perilla frutescens	5 fen
桔梗	jié gěng	Root of Platycodon grandiflorum	1 qian
甘草	gān cǎo	Root of Glycyrrhiza uralensis	1 qian

The decoction shall be taken warm. Five fen of **bái jiè zǐ** is added for patients with phlegm.

疳症

此脾熱而因乎心熱也，遂至口中流涎。若不平其心火，則脾火更旺，濕熱上蒸而口涎不能止。方用：

蘆薈、桑白皮各壹錢，黃連、薄荷、半夏各參分，茯苓貳錢，甘草壹分，水煎服。

此心脾兩清之聖藥也，引火下行而疳自去矣。

Malnutrition

Spleen heat is ascribed to heart heat, which in turn leads to dribbling. If heart heat is not pacified, spleen fire will be more effulgent and dampness-heat would steam upward so that the dribbling can in no way be stopped. Formula:

蘆薈 lú huì Aloe vera L. var. chinensis (Haw.) Berg. 1 qian

桑白皮	sāng bái pí	Root bark of Morus alba L.	1 qian
黃連	huáng lián	Rhizome of Coptis chinensis	3 fen
薄荷	bò hé	Plant of Mentha Haplocalyx	3 fen
半夏	bàn xià	Rhizome of Pinellia ternata	3 fen
茯苓	fú líng	Dried fungus of Poria cocos	2 qian
甘草	gān căo	Root of Glycyrrhiza uralensis	1 fen

This is a sovereign remedy for clearing both heart and spleen. It conducts fire downward and the malnutrition is gone by itself.

口疳流水口爛神方

黃柏貳錢，人參壹錢，共為細末，敷口內，一日三次即愈。

此方用黃柏去火，人參健脾，大人用之亦效。

A Sovereign Remedy for Oral Erosion, Dribbling and Ulcer of Oral Cavity

Grind two qian of **huáng băi** and one qian of **rén shén** into fine powder, apply the powder to patient's oral cavity for three times a day and it cures.

This formula for *oral erosion*[145], dribbling and ulcer of oral cavity uses **huáng bǎi** to eliminate fire and **rén shén** to fortify spleen. The formula is applicable to adults.

疳症瀉痢眼障神效方

石決明壹兩醋煆，蘆薈、川芎、白蒺藜、胡黃連、五靈脂、細辛、谷精草各伍錢，甘草叁錢，菊花肆錢，豬肝去筋，搗爛為丸如桐子大，每服貳拾伍丸。不拘時，米湯下。

A Magic Remedy for Malnutrition, Dysenteric Diarrhea and Eyesight Obstacle

石決明 shí jué míng Concha Haliotidis (Abalone shell) (processed with vinegar) 1 liang

蘆薈 lú huìAloe vera L. var. chinensis (Haw.) Berg. 5 qian

川芎 chuān xiōng Root of Ligusticum wallichii 5 qian

白蒺藜 bái jí lí Fruit of Puncturevine Caltrop 5 qian

胡黃連 hú huáng lián Rhizome of Figwortflower Picrorhiza 5 qian

145 *Oral erosion:* a condition marked by multiple spots of erosion on the buccal mucosa.

五靈脂 wǔ líng zhīDung of Complex-toothed Flying Squirrel 5 qian

細辛 xì xīn Complete plant of Asarum heteropoides 5 qian

谷精草 gǔ jīng cǎo Flower of Pipewort 5 qian

甘草 gān cǎo Root of Glycyrrhiza uralensis 3 qian

菊花 jú huā Flower of Chrysanthemum morafolii 4 qian

Remove the veins of **zhū líng** and pound it into pulps to be prepared into pills in size of tung-oil tree seed. Take twenty-five pieces each time with thin rice gruel. The time of intake is not set.

瘧疾

方用：

柴胡陸分，白朮、茯苓、歸身各壹錢，白芍壹錢伍分，半夏、青皮、厚樸各伍分，水煎成，露一宿，再溫與服。

熱多者，加人參、黃耆各伍分；寒多者，加乾薑參分；痰多者，加白芥子壹錢；夜熱加何首烏、熟地各貳錢，日發者不用加；腹痛加檳榔參分。

Malaria

Formula:

柴胡 chái hú Root of Bupleurum chinense 6 fen

白术 bái zhú Rhizome of Atractylodes macrocephala 1 qian
茯苓 fú líng Dried fungus of Poria cocos 1 qian
歸身 guī shēn Main root of Angelica polimorpha 1 qian
白芍 bái sháo Root of Paeonia lactiflora 1 qian 5 fen
半夏 bàn xià Rhizome of Pinellia ternata 5 fen
青皮 qīng pí Immature peel of Citrus reticulata 5 fen
厚樸 hòu pò Bark of Magnolia officinalis 5 fen

The decoction shall be set aside overnight and warmed before taking.

Five fen of **rén shén** and five fen of **huáng qí** are added for patients with excessive heat; Three fen of **gān jiāng** is added for patients of excessive cold; One qian of **bái jiè zǐ** is added for those with excessive phlegm; Two qian of **hé shǒu wū** and two qian of **shú dì** are added for those with elevated temperature during night but not to add anything for those with elevated temperature during daytime; Three fen of **bīng láng** shall be added for those with abdomeninal pains.

便蟲

方用：

榧子伍個去殼，甘草參分，米飯為丸。服二次，則蟲化為水矣。

Worm Stool

Formula:

榧子去殼 fěi zi Seed of Torreya grandis Fort.ex Lindl. (without shell) 5 pieces

甘草 gān cǎo Root of Glycyrrhiza uralensis 3 fen

Make pills with cooked rice and prepare into two dosages. Worms will be turned into water after the second dose.

積蟲

方用：

史君子去殼炒、榧子各拾箇去殼，檳榔、甘草各壹錢，米飯為丸，如桐子大，每服十丸，二日蟲出，五日全愈。

Worm Stagnation

Formula:

史君子去殼炒 shǐ jūn zǐ Fruit of Rangooncreeper (without shell and fried) 10 pieces

榧子去殼 fěi zi Seed of Torreya grandis Fort.ex Lindl. (without shell) 10 pieces

檳榔 bīng láng Fruit of Areca catechu 1 qian

甘草 gān cǎo Root of Glycyrrhiza uralensis 1 qian

Make pills with cooked rice in size of tung-oil tree seed, take ten pieces each time and the worm will be out in two days. It cures in five days.

痘症回毒或疔腫

方用：

銀花伍錢，人參貳錢，甘草、元參貳錢，水煎服。

Pernicious Influence of Smallpox or Deep-rooted Boil

Formula:

銀花 yín huā Flower of Lonicera japonica 5 qian

人參 rén shén Root of Panax ginseng 2 qian

甘草 gān cǎo Root of Glycyrrhiza uralensis 2 qian

元參 yuán shēn Root of Scrophularia ningpoensis 2 qian

痘瘡壞症已黑

痘瘡壞證已黑者，人將棄之，藥下喉即活。方用：

人參叁錢，陳皮、荊芥各壹錢，蟬退伍分，元參、當歸各貳錢，水煎服。

此乃元氣虛而火不能發也，故用人參以補元氣；元參去浮游之火；陳皮去痰開胃，則參無礙，而相得益彰；荊芥以發之，又能引火以歸經；當歸生新去舊，消瘀血；蟬退解毒除風。世人何知此妙法。初起時不可服，必壞證乃可服。

Deteriorated Case of Smallpox

Children with deteriorated case of small box turns black in color, and parents are going to give up. However, they will recover soon after taking the decoction of this formula:

人參	rén shén	Root of Panax ginseng	3 qian
陳皮	chén pí	Peel of Citrus reticulata	1 qian
荊芥	jīng jiè	Leaf of Schizonepeta tenuifolia	1 qian
蟬退	chán tuì	Exuviae of Cicada	5 fen
元參	yuán shēn	Root of Scrophularia ningpoensis	2 qian
當歸	dāng guī	Root of Angelica polimorpha	2 qian

The case is due to compressed fire of source qi4 deficiency. Therefore, **rén shén** is used to tonfiy source qi4, **yuán shēn** is used to eliminate floating fire and **chén pí** is used to dispel phlegm and increase appetite, so that the former two medicinals are of no obstacle to but bring out the best in each other. **Jīng jiè** is to develop it, and conducts fire back to its own meridian. **Dāng guī** engenders the new, dispels the old and resolves static blood. **Chán tuì** detoxifies and dispels wind. What a wonderful formula! But this formula is not applicable to the onset sphere of smallpox, but to those deteriorated cases.

急慢風

急、慢驚風，三、六、九日一切風俱治。

陳膽星、雄黃、硃砂、人參、茯苓、天竺黃、鉤籐、牛黃、麝香、川鬱金、柴胡、青皮、甘草。為細末，煎膏為丸如莞豆大，真金一張為衣，陰乾勿洩氣，薄荷湯磨服。

Acute and Chronic Infantile Convulsion

This formula treats all sorts of infantile convulsion, whether acute, chronic, three-day, six-day or nine-day convulsion:

陳膽星	chén dǎn xīng	Preserved Arisaema with bile
雄黃	xióng huáng	Realgar
朱砂	zhū shā	Cinnabar
人參	rén shén	Root of Panax ginseng

茯苓	fú líng	Dried fungus of Poria cocos
天竺黄	tiān zhú huáng	Sap of Bambusa textilis McClure
鉤籐	gōu téng	Stem of Ramulus Uncariae cum Uncis
牛黃	niú huáng	Powder of cow bezoar
麝香	shè xiāng	Dried secretion from the musk pod of Moschus moschiferus
川鬱金	chuān yù jīn	Root of Curcuma aromatica
柴胡	chái hú	Root of Bupleurum chinense
青皮	qīng pí	Immature peel of Citrus reticulata
甘草	gān cǎo	Root of Glycyrrhiza uralensis

Grind the medicinals into fine powder, decoct into paste to make pills in size of garden pea. Wrap the pills into a piece of gold foil to dry in shade so as to not let go of qi4. Grind the pills for intake with *Bo He Tang* [pinyin: bò he tāng, 薄荷湯, Decoction of plant of Mentha Haplocalyx].

治火丹神方

絲瓜子、元參各壹兩，柴胡、升麻各壹錢，當歸伍錢，水煎服。又方：

升麻、青蒿、黄耆各叁錢，元參壹兩，乾葛參兩，水煎服。

此二方詳火證，小兒用之亦效，故又出之。此方妙在用青蒿，肝胃之火俱平，又佐以群藥重劑，而火安有不滅者乎？

A Magic Formula for Erysipelas

絲瓜子 sī guā zǐ Seed of Luffa cylindrica(L.) Roem. 1 liang

元參 yuán shēn Root of Scrophularia ningpoensis 1 liang

柴胡 chái hú Root of Bupleurum chinense 1 qian

升麻 shēng má Rhizome of Cimifuga foetida 1

q i a n

當歸 dāng guī Root of Angelica polimorpha 5 qian

Another formula:

升麻 shēng má Rhizome of Cimifuga foetida 3 qian

青蒿 qīng hāo Foliage of Artemisiae Apiacceae 3 qian

黃耆 huáng qí Root of Astragalus membranaceus 3 qian

元參 yuán shēn Root of Scrophularia ningpoensis 1 liang

乾葛 gān gē Dried root of Pueraria lobata 3 liang

The two formulae stipulated again, specify in treating *erysipelas*[146] and are applicable to children as well. The genius of the second formula consists in its use of **qīng hāo**, which pacifies both liver and stomach fire. Assisted by heavy dosage of other medicinals, how can the fire not be extinguished?

146 *erysipelas*: an acute infection of the skin marked by intense local redness

www.ingramcontent.com/pod-product-compliance
Lightning Source LLC
Chambersburg PA
CBHW031818170526
45157CB00001B/101